Macrobiotics Beyond Food

By the same author:

Macrobiotics: Yesterday and Today

292 pp., 7-1/4×10-1/4 inches, 54 black-and-white
photos, bibliography, index. (1985)

LCCC 84–81358
ISBN 0–87040–611–6

Macrobiotics Beyond Food

A Guide to Health and Well-Being

Ronald E. Kotzsch, Ph.D.

Japan Publications, Inc.

Published by JAPAN PUBLICATIONS, INC., Tokyo and New York

Distributors:
UNITED STATES: *Kodansha International/USA, Ltd., through Harper & Row, Publishers, Inc., 10 East 53rd Street, New York, New York 10022.* SOUTH AMERICA: *Harper & Row, Publishers, Inc., International Department.* CANADA: *Fitzhenry & Whiteside Ltd., 195 Allstate Parkway, Markham, Ontario, L3R 4T8.* MEXICO AND CENTRAL AMERICA: *HARLA S. A. de C. V., Apartado 30–546, Mexico 4, D. F.* BRITISH ISLES: *Premier Book Marketing Ltd., 1 Gower Street, London WC1E 6HA.* EUROPEAN CONTINENT: *European Book Service PBD, Strijkviertel 63, 3454 PK de Meern, The Netherlands.* AUSTRALIA AND NEW ZEALAND: *Bookwise International, 1 Jeanes Street, Beverley, South Australia 5007.* THE FAR EAST AND JAPAN: *Japan Publications Trading Co., Ltd., 1–2–1, Sarugaku-cho, Chiyoda-ku, Tokyo 101.*

First edition: July 1988

LCCC No. 86–81324
ISBN 0–87040–674–4

Printed in U.S.A.

Foreword

Over twenty years ago I first met Aveline and Michio Kushi and discovered Macrobiotics. I began to study its philosophy and to incorporate its practices, especially those regarding diet, into my life. Since then I have continued to study and practice Macrobiotics (albeit in an idiosyncratic and sporadic way). I have been a student and associate of the Kushi's since that time, and have studied also with Herman and Cornellia Aihara, with Mrs. Lima Ohsawa, and many other distinguished teachers. From 1977 through 1981 I immersed myself in the life and work of George Ohsawa, the leading modern teacher of Macrobiotics, and produced a Ph. D. thesis on "George Ohsawa and the Japanese Religious Tradition."

When I began Macrobiotics I thought that it was a diet aimed at physical health. I soon realized that while it includes a diet Macrobiotics is really a way of life. I realized as well that Macrobiotics is concerned with the health not of just the physical body, but of the whole human being, in its emotional, intellectual and other dimensions.

During those years I was involved in various other activities. I was a graduate student (in World Religions at Harvard and in Japanese Culture at Kyoto National University); a cab driver and natural foods retailer (in Chicago); a prep school teacher (of Philosophy and Religion) and athletic coach (of Cross Country and Track); an instructor for Outward Bound (at the Dartmouth College Center of the Hurricane Island Outward Bound); a college professor (of Religion at Hampden-Sydney College of Virginia); and magazine journalist (as a writer for *East West*). I was also a student of Hatha Yoga, a serious long distance runner, and bicyclist.

From these other, non-Macrobiotic activities, I learned a great deal about health and about how to cultivate it. I realized early on that what I learned—as an academic, wilderness trip leader, teacher, journalist, cab driver and athlete—was in fact part of

Macrobiotics. This was no original discovery of course. I had
been taught by Mr. Kushi (through example, lecture and conversation) and by Mr. Ohsawa (through the many books of his
which I had read) that Macrobiotics is a way of life in harmony
with the universal order, and thus involves everything we think,
do and say. It took me a while however to be able to really hear
and understand this.

In 1978 I began teaching at the Kushi Institute in Boston,
and used in my classes there the concept of "Macrobiotics Beyond Food." Macrobiotics includes a diet, I pointed out, but it
is not only a diet. It is a full way of life which involves the conscious and careful cultivation of each area of life. Just as we
carefully nourish and exercise the physical body, we must feed
and strengthen the other aspects of our humanity, from aesthetic
to spiritual. I developed this idea using material from the existing
Macrobiotic literature and from my personal studies and
experience.

In 1981 I began to give the resulting seminar in other places
in the United States and in Europe. Since then I have presented
"Macrobiotics Beyond Food" more times than I can remember.
I have lectured in a variety of venues—in a magnficent conven-
tion center in Innsbruck, Austria; in a damp, cramped basement
in Edinburgh, Scotland; under a canopy of blue sky and swaying
pines in the Sierra Nevada mountains of California; and in
a lecture room in Tokyo, where the fluorescent lights were so
numerous and bright that I felt in danger of sunstroke. These
talks were generally well received. At least no member of the
audience became ill or passed away during them, and most of
those attending remained present and conscious until the end.
Boos, hisses and threats on my life were at a minimum. More
than a few people came up afterward and said that in the
process Macrobiotics had become much broader and deeper for
them.

Two years ago with the encouragement and support of Japan
Publications I decided to render these lectures into book form.
My motivation was twofold. First I wanted to make the ideas
available to a wider audience. Second I wanted to liberate myself

from having to give the lectures anymore. By that time, if I had been awakened at midnight, hung upside down by my toes, and hosed with cold water, I probably could have intoned the whole *spiel* without skipping a word. I was ready to move on to new issues.

Turning a series of lectures into a book has proved to be interesting and difficult. Like any worthwhile task—climbing a mountain, running a marathon, keeping a woman happy—it has required 20 percent more time, energy and imagination than I expected it would. The result of this effort is *Macrobiotics Beyond Food: A Guide to Health and Well-Being*. The book is derivative, eclectic, personal, idiosyncratic, tentative, and practical.

Macrobiotics Beyond Food is derivative in that its basic outlook is based on the teachings of George Ohsawa and Michio Kushi. Both men have profoundly influenced my ideas and my life.

This book is eclectic because I have drawn on various other sources. Most of these, while not expressly Macrobiotic, share its philosophical perspective and its aims. These sources include my own Lutheran-Christian background and faith; the various world religious traditions I have studied; and other philosophies and disciplines which I have found useful, particularly the Anthroposophy of German philosopher Rudolph Steiner (1861–1925), and the educational views of Outward Bound founder Kurt Hahn (1895–1980). On occasion I have even resorted to common sense.

It is personal and idiosyncratic because it is my own interpretation of Macrobiotics. While I presume to speak for the Macrobiotic community, I ultimately am speaking only for myself.

It is tentative in that it is only an initial attempt at describing Macrobiotics as a comprehensive way of life. It does not pretend to contain the definitive view on any of the issues raised. It is meant largely to stimulate further thought, study and discussion.

And finally this book is practical in that its principal aim is to provide simple, practical suggestions for creating a healthy and happy life.

A book seems to have a single creator, but in fact has many. And many people through their encouragement and help have shared in the making of *Macrobiotics Beyond Food*. They include:

- My mother, Martha Koetzsch, who in the simplicity and richness of her life and the generosity of her spirit manifests the ideals of Macrobiotics.
- My sister Anita and her family—Edward, Christine, and Ronny—who are always absolutely generous in their love and laughter.
- The Rev. Jackson M. Smith of the New North Church in Hingham, Massachusetts, who as a friend and supporter knows no equal.
- The members of the New North Church who have amiably tolerated my literary squatterdom these many years.
- Aveline and Michio Kushi and their family who have treated me as one of their own for over two decades.
- My professors and fellow students at the Center for the Study of World Religions, Harvard University, from whom I have learned much, in the classroom and outside of it.
- My students and fellow instructors at Outward Bound, where I learned to treasure challenge and the outdoors.
- Mr. Iwao Yoshizaki, president of Japan Publications, and Mr. Yoshiro Fujiwara, the company's American representative, who have been so patient and kind in encouraging and waiting for the birth of this book.
- John and Sarah Paino who are special friends and did much to help during these past, often trying, months.
- Stevan Goldin, my perceptive, astute, and careful editor and proofreader.
- Steve Cohen and Pauline Kenney, my meticulous final proofreaders.

I thank all these people, as well as my many other benefactors.

I must apologize in advance for my failure to use only gender-inclusive language. Though raised in a more sexist era and educated at an all-male and, at that time, sexist university, I have had most of my sexism pommeled out of me by several feminist friends. Thus I sympathize with the use of language that includes both sexes on equal terms. And I happily use "person" and "humanity" rather than "man" and "mankind."

However, as a writer concerned with style I cannot bring myself to use the "he/she," "his/her," and "him/her" usages, as in the sentence "Every human being should take good care of his/her body." They are to me very awkward and distracting. Therefore I usually use "he," "his," and 'him," when such a gender-inclusive construction might be more correct. Please let it be known that I do so intending that both sexes be equally denoted, and with respectful apologies to all offended.

RONALD E. KOTZSCH
Church Office
The New North Church
Hingham, Massachusetts
3 December 1987

Contents

Introduction

The word *health* comes from the Anglo-Saxon word *hal*, which means "whole." Health, usually defined as "the absence of physical pain and disease," is a major human concern. Next to it, all the other important issues in human life, such as wealth, love, and power, pale into relative insignificance. However otherwise blessed we may be, if we must struggle daily with the pain of arthritis, migraine headaches, or a bad back, it is difficult or impossible to be happy. On the other hand, however poor and humble, if we can live without pain or dysfunction we have the foundation for a happy and satisfying life.

Unfortunately, maintaining this state of "wholeness" has been a problem since the beginning of recorded history and before. There is evidence of *disease*, "the loss of ease," among our prehistoric ancestors. And in every civilization from ancient times to the present, a host of maladies have plagued humankind. Medicine, the art of gaining and preserving health, and the physicians and healers who practice it, have played an important role in every culture. Today, in our modern society, illness is common, almost universal, and the medical enterprise continues. There are physicians, clinics, and hospitals all over the world, particularly in the developed nations. These are a testimony to our desire for health and to our continuing failure to realize it. Hospitals, after all, are filled with sick people, not with healthy ones.

About thirty years ago a Japanese philosopher named Yukikazu Sakurazawa (better known as George Ohsawa) arrived in the West and began to teach what he claimed to be a sure path to health. Calling this *Macrobiotics*, or "the great art of life," Ohsawa presented ideas which challenged common assumptions about health, sickness, and medicine.

Ohsawa rejected, for example, the negative and one-dimensional definition of health as the "absence of disease."

He maintained rather that health is a positive and multidimensional condition, which includes both physical and psychological aspects. True health according to Ohsawa consists of:

- consistent and high physical energy;
- the ability to fall asleep easily and to awake after a few hours totally refreshed;
- a hearty appetite for simple, nourishing food, and for sex;
- a positive and happy frame of mind, even in the midst of difficulties;
- a good memory;
- clarity and speed in thought and action; and
- a profound gratitude for the gift of life.

Ohsawa considered such a state of health to be the natural birthright of every human being. It is not an unattainable ideal but a practical possibility. We can indeed realize it. And whether we do so or not depends on ourselves and how we live. The human being is a creature of nature and if he lives in harmony with nature he can gain and maintain health. Thus, Ohsawa challenged the idea that illness is an inescapable fact of human life and that health is the fleeting privilege of the young and the lucky. He challenged as well, the assumption that we have little control over our health, that illness strikes us as innocent victims, randomly, or by the inscrutable will of God.

Ohsawa also taught that daily food is a very important factor in human health and sickness. A diet in harmony with the natural order, he maintained, is the necessary foundation of health. It will prevent and cure illness. A diet violating this order leads inevitably to sickness and unhappiness. Ohsawa recommended a way of eating in which whole cereal grains are the primary food, and are supplemented by beans, local and seasonal vegetables and fruits, and by seeds, nuts, and small amounts of animal food, usually fish. He warned against refined foods such as white sugar and white flour, against foods containing large percentages of animal fat and protein (red meat, dairy foods), and against all chemicalized and industrially fabricated, processed foods. Here again Ohsawa was going against established thought. The medical and popular wisdom of the day held that a "well-balanced" diet must include meat and dairy products, and that as long as one ate from "the four basic food groups" (meat, dairy, starchy foods, and vegetables and fruits), food was not ordinarily a factor in illness or recovery. This view held also that the surest, indeed only, medical treatment was based on drugs and surgery.

In the ten years prior to his death in 1966, Ohsawa was very active in Europe and the United States. He attracted a dedicated but small following. The Macrobiotic view of health, sickness, and healing was too radical for most people. Moreover, Ohsawa presented these ideas in the context of a Taoist *Yin-Yang* philosophy. This approach gave his teachings an exotic and alien quality, attractive to some but obscure and upsetting to many. Also, the particular foods Ohsawa recommended—brown rice, *miso* soup (made from fermented soybean paste), sea vegetables, *daikon* radish, lotus root, and the like—added to this strangeness. And Ohsawa championed the stricter forms of the diet, saying that *Diet Number Seven* (consisting only of whole grains, preferably brown rice) was the most effective form of the Macrobiotic regime. In *Zen Macrobiotics*, his first book in English, Ohsawa wrote that if carefully observed for ten days, Diet Number Seven could cure almost any disease. Thus in the early 1960s, Macrobiotics was generally viewed as a radical, food-oriented Japanese cult.

After Ohsawa's death, several of his Japanese disciples, already living in America, continued his work. These included Michio and Aveline Kushi and Herman and Cornellia Aihara. The movement continued and grew, and in the past two decades the Macrobiotic diet has become widely known and practiced in America and around the world.

There are several reasons for this growth, which continues yet today, slowly but steadily. One is that the public's attitudes about health and diet have changed, and Ohsawa's ideas are not considered so radical as they once were. The Macrobiotic view of health as positive and multidimensional; of the responsibility of each person for his own health; and of the importance of food as a factor in health have all become widely, if not universally accepted.

This acceptance has been due in part to the efforts of the Kushis, Aiharas, and other Macrobiotic teachers. In greater part perhaps, it is because the holistic health movement (of which Macrobiotics is a part) has been promoting many of these same ideas (from various perspectives) since the early 1970's. Besides, research carried on within the medical and scientific establishment has confirmed many of Ohsawa's ideas about food. It has shown that:

- Diet is indeed a crucial factor in health.
- Foods rich in complex carbohydrates and fibre (whole grains, beans, seeds, fresh vegetables and fruits) promote health.
- Foods rich in animal fats and proteins (red meat, eggs, cheese), or in simple carbohydrates (white flour, white sugar), may contribute to illness.

Also, Kushi (based in Boston), and Aihara (based in California), while honoring the core and the spirit of Ohsawa's teachings, have moderated the Macrobiotic dietary recommendations. Both realized years ago that most people, and especially young Americans raised on hamburgers, French fries, soft drinks, ice cream, and recreational drugs, cannot thrive on a diet of brown rice and miso soup. Hence they began to advise a broader, more varied diet. Kushi, since the early 1970's, has promoted *The Standard Macrobiotic Diet* as a general guideline for those wishing to improve their health. This regime consists of 50 percent whole grains or whole-grain products, 10 percent beans, 25 percent cooked vegetables, 5 percent soup, and the balance in seeds, nuts, seasonal, fresh and dried fruits, and fish. And meanwhile, Aveline Kushi, Cornellia Aihara, and a host of other Macrobiotic cooks and teachers of cooking, have developed a broad and delicious Macrobiotic cuisine. Incorporating traditional European and American foods and methods of preparation, this cuisine appeals to most palates. The rigorous Diet Number Seven is seldom mentioned or practiced, and is regarded mainly as a kind of fast, to be done in special circumstances, for a short time.

Another factor in the spread of Macrobiotics is that, even in this moderate form, it has proven to be an effective therapy for various illnesses. People suffering from arthritis, diabetes, heart disease, obesity, asthma, and even cancer, have been greatly helped by the Macrobiotic diet. Some of the more dramatic cases have received attention from the mass media. The most notable is that of Dr. Anthony Satillaro, a physician who cured his cancer with the help of Macrobiotic eating, and who wrote a book, *Recalled By Life* (Houghton Mifflin, Boston, 1980), about his experience.

In any case, Macrobiotics today is widely known and there are thousands of people, perhaps hundreds-of-thousands, in North and South America, Europe, Australia and New Zealand, and in many parts of Asia and Africa who are eating some form of the Macrobiotic diet. Nevertheless, there remains a basic and almost universal misunderstanding about Macrobiotics. Most people, including many of those eating according to Macro-biotic principles, think that Macrobiotics is only a diet, that Macrobiotics and the Macrobiotic way of eating are the same thing. This view is both inaccurate and dangerous.

It is inaccurate because Macrobiotics and the Macrobiotic diet are two distinct, if related, things. Macrobiotics, in itself, is a "practical philosophy." As such, it includes a philosophy, or view of the universe, and of human nature and destiny. It includes also a "practice," or way of living, based on this phi-losophy and purporting to lead to health and happiness. Because eating is an important part of human life, the Macrobiotic way of life involves a diet, or more accurately, an approach to food. But it involves various other practices as well. Also based on the Macrobiotic philosophy, and also aiming at human health, some of these practices, such as proper exercise and the use of natural fabrics in clothing, concern the physical body. But many are related to the other dimensions of the human being—emotional, intellectual, social, moral, and spiritual. Hence diet, while an important part of the Macrobiotic way of life, is only one aspect of it. Macrobiotics is "the great art of living" not "the great art of eating."

The view of Macrobiotics as a diet is dangerous because it can mislead those seeking health and well-being. Certainly food is a key factor in our lives. It directly affects our physical condition and is an important influence in any recovery from illness. It plays a role as well in our emotional and psychological lives. But diet is only one piece of the puzzle. Proper eating alone cannot prevent nor cure illness. It alone can give us neither health nor happiness. What we do in each domain of life is also important, for our physical health and for our general well-being. A person's emotional, moral, psychological, and spiritual condition all affect the origin and course of any illness. Thus, to be truly healthy and happy, we must devote time and energy to cultivating each aspect of life. We must eat in harmony with the order of the universe, but we must also arrange every other aspect of our life according to it.

Of course, neither George Ohsawa nor his successors intended to present Macrobiotics simply as a diet. Ohsawa made clear that Macrobiotics is a way of life founded on a view of the universe. He often complained that he was weary of talking about food and that he much preferred to discuss other topics, such as art, ethics, politics, and religion. In fact, his emphasis on Diet Number Seven in his latter years may have come from a desire to make the issue of food as simple and straightforward (and quickly dealt with) as possible.

Kushi, Aihara, and other leading teachers have also stressed the breadth of Macrobiotics. Kushi has treated a wide range of issues, from agriculture to world peace, from sexuality to spiritual practices. Aihara's favorite topics include personal relationships and the attainment of individual peace of mind. Nevertheless, the perception of Macrobiotics as a diet persists. The teachings and recommendations about areas other than food tend to get lost among the recipes for carrot pie and vegetable dumplings.

Macrobiotics Beyond Food is an attempt to remedy this misunderstanding of Macrobiotics as just a diet. It is an attempt to present Macrobiotics as a comprehensive and coherent way of life.

Macrobiotics Beyond Food is organized very simply, using a sevenfold division of the human being. Mr. Ohsawa used this schema in discussing various topics such as the *Seven Levels of Human Judgment*, and the *Seven Levels of Sickness*. According to it, the human being is made up of seven distinct, but interrelated dimensions or "bodies"—the physical, aesthetic, emotional, intellectual, social, ideological, and the spiritual. The totality of our life therefore has seven areas corresponding to these seven bodies.

Chapter 1, "The Heart of the Macrobiotic Artichoke," presents the Macrobiotic world view in terms of seven key ideas. Chapters 2 through 8 deal in turn with the physical, aesthetic, emotional, intellectual, social, ideological, and spiritual areas of life. Each explores how, with the Macrobiotic philosophy as a basis, we can cultivate "wholeness" in a particular area of life. Chapter 9 deals with the issue of illness and healing. And a brief Conclusion reviews some crucial points.

Macrobiotics Beyond Food is written for the person totally unfamiliar with Macrobiotics, for the beginner in his early practice and for the longtime practitioner as well. By making clear the philosophy and spirit of Macrobiotics, and by demonstrating that this philosophy and spirit can enrich every area of life, it will benefit, I hope, all those who read it.

1. The Heart of
the Macrobiotic Artichoke

Macrobiotics is an extreme, fad diet of Japanese
origin, which in ideal form consists entirely of un-
polished or "brown" rice. It is extremely dangerous
and can lead to malnutrition and death.
A nutrition textbook, 1985

Macrobiotics is a universal path to perfect health,
total freedom, and eternal happiness.
George Ohsawa (1893–1966)

Our focus in this book is the practice of Macrobiotics "beyond
food"—how in areas of life other than diet we can cultivate
health and well-being. Before we address that topic we must
look at the philosophy of Macrobiotics, the ideas about the
universe, human nature, and human destiny which lie behind
Macrobiotic practice. And we must examine the Macrobiotic
approach to food. Then we will be ready to look at Macrobiotics as a "way of life," which includes every aspect of human
life, from the physical to the spiritual.

This conceptual basis at which we must first look consists of
seven ideas which together may be called "The Heart of the
Macrobiotic Artichoke." Amidst the many varied ideas promulgated in the name of Macrobiotics, they are essential and
central. The first is metaphysical, attempting to explain the
origin and working of the universe. The second is anthropo-
logical, giving a view of human nature. The third defines human
health, and the fourth affirms the feasibility of health and our
own role in realizing it. The fifth and sixth concern the importance of food and the proper way to choose it. And the seventh
asserts the necessity of a way of life "beyond food." The seven
elements of "The Heart of the Macrobiotic Artichoke" are as
follows:

1. The universe is an infinitely diverse but monistic and integrated organism constantly in flux according to dialectical and orderly patterns. (Please do not be alarmed. This will be explained immediately—and in English.)

According to Ohsawa, the single reality in the universe is "the ocean of infinity." It is an undifferentiated cosmic oneness, infinite and eternal, which creates and contains within it all phenomena. Various cultures, referring to the same absolute, have given it different names—such as Yahweh, God, Allah, Brahman, the Tao, Shunyata, and The Great Spirit. This absolute is beyond space and time, and all duality. Within it there is no light nor darkness, no growth nor decay. Ohsawa also refers to it as "infinite expansion," "the world of Spirit," "the seventh Heaven," and "the domain of endless freedom, eternal happiness, and perfect justice."

According to Ohsawa, the creation of the finite world from the Infinite is a process which has been going on, without beginning, in the past, is going on now, and will continue forever in the future. It commences with the intersection of streams of energy moving at infinite speed in every direction. As two currents of water come together and form a whirlpool, the two streams intersect and create a contracting, centripetal spiral of energy. This vortex is three-dimensional, having depth as well as height and breadth.

This centripetal vortex creates a contractive energy, which Ohsawa, using traditional Oriental terminology, calls *Yang*. When it reaches the central point, and can contract no further, it begins to expand. A centrifugal spiral is formed, creating an expansive energy called *Yin*. Thus, within an undifferentiated Infinity, two finite and dialectical or opposing poles are formed. Ohsawa called this realm, in which only Yin and Yang exist, the "sixth Heaven," or the "realm of bipolarity." From the interaction of Yin and Yang is born the realm of space, time, and energy. In this "fifth Heaven" appear light, radiation, and electromagnetic energy. These are somewhat "contracted" forms of the cosmic principles of Yin and Yang.

The "fourth Heaven," proceeding from the fifth, and a slightly contracted form of it, is the realm of preatomic particles. These include the neutrons, protons, and electrons which are the building blocks of the atoms. These particles are contracted and more slowly moving manifestations of the energy world, and are controlled by magnetism.

The next level, that of the chemical elements, is the first stage of the visible material world, and is controlled by electricity. The preatomic particles form into elements, and these form the phenomena of the inanimate world—stars (our sun one among them), planets (our earth one among them), and on this earth, the soil, atmosphere, and water.

This "third Heaven" gives birth to the first stage of organic life which is plants. From the soil, air, and water emerge the countless forms of vegetative life, which grow, reproduce, and die.

This "second Heaven" of plants produces the "first Heaven," that of animate life. This world of microorganisms, insects, reptiles, fish, and mammals emerges from and is nourished by the plant kingdom. Like plants, these organisms grow, reproduce, decline, and die. But unlike plants, they are capable of movement and of learning new patterns of behavior.

The final manifestation of the animate kingdom, and in effect, the culmination of the whole process of creation, is the human being. Part of the animal realm, the human being also transcends it. Capable of understanding the universe and his place in it, the human being is the perfect manifestation of Infinity in the material realm. He is that being in which Infinity can become perfectly aware of itself.

Ohsawa presented this view of the universe in a schematic fashion, which he called *The Spiral of Creation*. (See figure 1.)

From this viewpoint, the universe is monistic, integrated, dialectical, harmonious, dynamic, and orderly.

It is monistic because all phenomena originate and exist within the single cosmic Absolute. Everything that exists, invisible and visible, inanimate and animate, is a manifestation of the Infinite Spirit.

It is integrated in that each of the "Heavens" is related to

Fig. 1 The Spiral of Creation. (Showing the seven levels of the evolution of the logarithmic spiral of the infinite universe.)

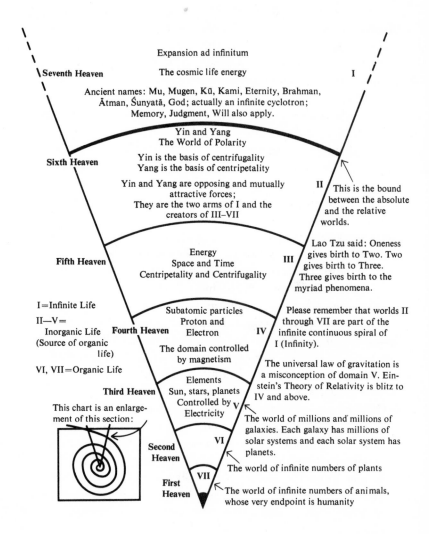

Expansion ad infinitum

Seventh Heaven   The cosmic life energy   I

Ancient names: Mu, Mugen, Kū, Kami, Eternity, Brahman, Ātman, Śunyatā, God; actually an infinite cyclotron; Memory, Judgment, Will also apply.

Yin and Yang
The World of Polarity

Sixth Heaven   Yin is the basis of centrifugality
Yang is the basis of centripetality

Yin and Yang are opposing and mutually   II   This is the bound
attractive forces;   between the absolute
They are the two arms of I and the   and the relative
creators of III–VII   worlds.

Lao Tzu said: Oneness
Energy   III   gives birth to Two. Two
Fifth Heaven   Space and Time   gives birth to Three.
Centripetality and Centrifugality   Three gives birth to the
myriad phenomena.

I=Infinite Life
Subatomic particles   Please remember that worlds II
II—V=   Proton and   through VII are part of the
Inorganic Life   Fourth Heaven   Electron   IV   infinite continuous spiral of
(Source of organic   I (Infinity).
life)   The domain controlled
by magnetism   The universal law of gravitation is
VI, VII=Organic Life   a misconception of domain V. Ein-
Elements   stein's Theory of Relativity is blitz to
Third Heaven   Sun, stars, planets   IV and above.
This chart is an enlarge-   Controlled by V
ment of this section: Electricity   The world of millions and millions of
galaxies. Each galaxy has millions of
VI   solar systems and each solar system has
Second   planets.
Heaven
The world of infinite numbers of plants
First   VII
Heaven   The world of infinite numbers of animals,
whose very endpoint is humanity

each of the other "Heavens." The whole forms a continuous spiral in which each realm is born of the one preceding and gives birth to the one following. Thus, every phenomena in the universe is related to every other phenomena of every realm, and all are related to the Infinite Spirit. Each leaf and ocean, child and star, is constantly influencing all that exists and is constantly being influenced by all that exists.

The universe is dialectical in that the Infinite Oneness manifests itself as two polar principles. One is contractive, active, and warm, and may be called the Yang or Male principle. The other is expansive, passive, and cool, and may be called the Yin or Female principle. The phenomenal world is created by, and operates according to, the interaction of Yin and Yang.

The universe is harmonious in that all apparent oppositions are in fact complementary. Every pair of antagonistic realities (Yin and Yang, light and darkness, day and night, energy and matter, man and woman, body and spirit, life and death, good and evil) forms a whole. Each phenomenon is born of, and in turn produces, its opposite. Neither can exist without the other.

The universe is dynamic in that everything is constantly changing. The only constant is change itself. Every electron, molecule, stone, flower, fish, mountain, and galaxy is in a continuous state of flux, changing into something else.

The universe is orderly in that all change occurs according to specific, predictable patterns or laws of change. These include:

- Yin attracts Yang. Yang attracts Yin.
- Yin repels Yin. Yang repels Yang.
- The force of attraction between two things is proportional to the difference of Yin and Yang between them. There is a strong attraction between extreme Yin and Yang, a lesser attraction between things that are moderately Yin and Yang.
- At the extreme, Yin becomes Yang, and Yang becomes Yin.

All phenomena in all realms of existence, operate according to these principles.

2. The human being, as a microcosm (small version) of the macrocosm, or universe, also is a diverse, but ultimately monistic and integrated organism. (Here again let us resort immediately to plain English.)

We human beings have several dimensions or "bodies." We have obviously a physical body, which is something like a biological machine. It takes in fuel, processes it to produce energy needed for its functioning and movement, and gives off waste products.

As part of this physical body we have sensory organs. These are sensitive to stimuli from the external environment—forms and colors, sounds, smells, tastes, heat, cold, and textures. These senses of sight, hearing, smell, taste, and touch comprise our "sensory" or "aesthetic body."

We have also an "emotional body" which responds to the world and our experiences. It registers joy, sadness, hope, despair, anger, compassion, love, hate, and many other emotions.

We also have a mind or "intellectual body." This intellectual faculty collects information about the world; it tries to see patterns of phenomena; it formulates laws, principles and ideas about the world and how it works.

In addition, each of us is interacting every day with other human beings, with animals, plants, and with the inanimate world. Our thoughts, words, and actions in relation to these other phenomena comprise our "social-moral body."

We have too an ideological faculty. Aware of ourselves as existing in an awesome and mysterious universe, we ask: "How did the universe come into being? How did humanity come into being? What is our final destiny?" and other ultimate questions. That part of us which poses these questions, which struggles with them, is our "ideological body."

Finally, we have a "spiritual body," a bit of the Infinite Spirit within us. This spirit yearns to be reunited with the cosmic

Oneness. It desires to transcend time and space and the limitations of the individual ego.

Thus, we have seven different "bodies," which are all
operative most of the time. At any given (waking) moment our
physical body is functioning; our sense organs are taking in
impressions; we are feeling some emotion, even if it is only
boredom; we have a thought pattern or idea in our mind; we
are interacting with something outside ourselves; we have an
opinion, expressed or unexpressed about the meaning or mean-
inglessness of life; and we have some sense of connection or
lack of connection with the source of reality.

These different bodies and the dimensions of life to which they
give rise, can be understood as profoundly interrelated or as
separate and unrelated. In fact, in the West, especially over the
past three centuries, we have tended to do the latter. The French
philosopher, René Descartes (1596–1650), asserted that the human body and the human mind are virtually unconnected. They
come tenuously together in the *pineal gland*, a small gland behind the eyes. Otherwise they operate separately according to
distinct laws and principles. This view helped promote the
dualistic attitude to body and mind which has dominated Western culture since. Hence, if we get physically sick we are likely
to seek out a physician; if we are mentally or spiritually disturbed we will probably seek out a psychiatrist or religious
counselor.

However, just as the kingdoms of nature all are part of a
continuous spiral and are all interrelated, so the bodies which
comprise the human being are interrelated. Each is an expanded
version of the one previous, and a contracted version of the one
following. Our emotional body, for example, is a somewhat
ethereal manifestation of our sensory body, and a more physical
manifestation of our intellectual body. Thus, while the various
bodies perform distinct functions, they actually comprise an
indivisible whole. Each is affecting all the others constantly.

For example, let us assume for a moment (only, alas) that you
have won twenty million dollars in the state lottery. This is a
strong positive, emotional experience, and you are probably

swept up in a transport of joy (unless of course your debts total forty million dollars). But each of your other bodies is simultaneously and strongly affected. You experience perhaps a great rush of physical energy. Suddenly everything in the world, even your mother-in-law, seems inexpressibly beautiful. Your head is filled with a racing kaleidoscope of plans and ideas about how to spend the money. You feel a warmth and love toward all creatures, and you may run around hugging trees. Any doubts you have had about the meaning of life immediately vanish. You may even feel at one with the universe, or at least with its local bank. Thus every body—physical, aesthetic, intellectual, social, ideological, and spiritual, as well as emotional—is profoundly affected. And if you were to receive a powerful negative emotional shock, again, all the bodies would be affected, but in a negative way. There are people whose hair has turned white overnight after the death of a loved one.

The lines of influence and connection go back and forth between all the different "bodies." Each is affecting all the others and each is being affected by all the others. Our human organism is like a spider's web with seven hubs or nodes in which are gathered the various strands of the web. Every node is connected to every other node. Thus, if there is any movement or change at a particular hub, then all the others are directly affected. Sometimes the changes are substantial and easily perceived. Often they are quite subtle and escape our conscious notice.

3. Human health or "wholeness" is the full and harmonious development of all the various human bodies. It is positive and multidimensional.

Even on the physical level, health is not merely the "absence of pain and dysfunction," but the positive development of the body's potential. It means, as Ohsawa pointed out, good sleep, good energy, and good appetite.

But health is the positive development in a balanced and harmonious way of each of the bodies, not only the physical. Thus the healthy person is aesthetically sensitive and creative; is cheerful and contented under all circumstances; is curious, has a good memory, and a positive way of thinking; is morally responsible; is concerned about the mystery of existence; and is striving toward, and to some degree realizing, a sense of oneness with a higher level of reality.

Sickness, as the absence of health, also is multidimensional. It is the absence of wholeness in any of the human bodies. Thus, to be blind to the beauty of the world; to be morose and discontent; to be uninterested and uninformed about the world; to be immoral in our dealings with other people and creatures; to be indifferent to the basic questions of life; and to feel lost and isolated in the universe; is to be as sick as if one had tuberculosis or a fatal heart disease.

4. We human beings have health as a natural birthright and we are totally responsible for our success or failure in realizing that birthright.

As infinity made manifest in the phenomenal world, we come into the world to realize our potential. We come to enjoy life, not just to suffer and die. Of course, perfect health and happiness is an ideal. As we approach it the laws of change propel us in the opposite direction. If we are spared a physical ailment for a long time we tend to abuse ourselves and make ourselves sick. The elation of a great accomplishment may be followed by depression. Some measure of pain, sickness, and sorrow is an inescapable part of human experience. But it is possible, on the continuum between health and sickness, to live closer to the positive pole than to the negative, and to be moving ever closer to it. It is possible to be healthy and happy.

Whether we in fact realize health or sickness depends entirely on ourselves. By our thoughts, words, and deeds we create ourselves and everything which happens to us.

For the most part, the operation of the law of cause and effect is fairly obvious. If I eat six rich meals a day and do not exercise I will get fat. If I practice the piano diligently I will become a skilled player; if I do not practice I will be a poor one. If I rob a bank, chances are I will wind up in jail.

However, many circumstances seem to be the result of blind

fate, or accident, or the arbitrary maliciousness of others. If I am born with leukemia, or into a family where I am abused and mistreated, how am I responsible? If I am walking by the scene of a robbery and am struck by a stray bullet, or if I am persecuted because of my race or religion, how am I responsible? In short, the world seems full of much apparently random and unmerited suffering. And it contains also many examples of what seems undeserved good fortune. How is a person born into wealth and comfort responsible for his circumstances?

The concepts of karma and reincarnation, basic to most Eastern religions and present in the Western religious tradition as well, address this issue. The law of karma, or action and reaction, is simply the application of Newton's Third Law of Physics (for every action there is an equal and opposite reaction) to the non-physical world. It maintains that everything we think, say, and do creates a certain energy and that this energy will come back to us. It may take months or years to return, and it may come back in another, unrecognizable form, but most certainly, "like bread cast upon the waters," it will return. Thus, the good or ill we do always comes back. Thus, what seems an accident or an arbitrary victimization is just the subtle but ineluctable working out of the law of karma.

The doctrine of reincarnation maintains that the human being evolves during many distinct lives, and that karma carries over from one life to the other. Thus, what we have thought, said, and done in one life can affect a subsequent life. We create and are responsible for even the circumstances of our birth, poor or privileged. We are the ultimate source of all the strikes and strokes of fortune.

Besides personal karma (karma generated by and returning to an individual), there is also family, communal, class, racial, national and planetary karma. This karma is created by the group and returns to the group, though not necessarily to the individuals who were originally involved. Thus, since we are all involved in some group karma, we may receive energy, good and bad, which we as individuals did not create. But since we choose our identity we are still responsible.

Karma and reincarnation notwithstanding, the concept of total responsibility is difficult to prove. Nevertheless, Macrobiotics as a path to health and happiness requires this concept. To accept responsibility is to become free to create our health and happiness.

For example, I can blame my sickness and unhappiness on my poor toilet training, on my second-rate education, on social prejudice, or on my wife's ill temper. However, I cannot change the past. Nor am I likely to change society or my wife. So I am forever locked in my miserable situation.

On the other hand, I can forget all negative and external factors of the past and present. I can acknowledge that I am totally responsible for myself and my life, past, present and future. Thus I become free to make myself and my life into what I wish, by changing the way I think, speak, and act. While I cannot easily alter other people or external circumstances, I can change myself. And upon that fact rests the promise of the Macrobiotic way of life.

5.   Diet is one, very important, factor in our achieving health.

Food is necessary to life. We begin eating shortly after birth and continue eating, three or four times a day, throughout our life. Food allows us to grow, to think and to act. Without food, life soon stops, and hence our appetite for it is consistent and strong.

What we eat obviously affects our physical health. Our food is digested and passes into the blood stream. There it nourishes and renews each cell of the body. The type and quality of the food affects the condition of the body, and from ancient times human beings have realized this. In Greece, China, India, and elsewhere, from early times to the present, food has been recognized as a key factor in maintaining health and in curing disease. Even modern allopathic medicine, which until recently ignored food as a factor in health, now is increasingly aware of its role in avoiding and in curing illness.

But food does not affect just our physical body. It influences each of our other bodies, from the aesthetic to the spiritual. Let us suppose that I am sitting with several friends chatting. Suddenly I take out a bottle of Glenlivet, ninety-proof unblended Scotch. I pour a stiff drink for each person and encourage them to enjoy it. I pour one for myself, drink it and pour another. Soon, noticeable changes begin to occur. My face flushes and my hand becomes a bit unsteady. I notice that the colors of the room have become very bright, and that the room is spinning around. I become, for no apparent reason, very happy, almost ecstatic. I have many brilliant but disordered insights about my life and the world at large. I start to interact with my friends in a new intimate way. I even give Charlie, who recently ran over my bicycle with his truck, a big hug. I start to muse on the great issues of life. I am overcome by a sense of oneness with my friends and with the larger world around me. Thus, because of the few drinks, every aspect of myself changes radically.

Now we think of alcohol as a drug because of the immediate and strong way in which it affects us. But alcohol is in effect a food. It is something we ingest, which is broken down, and which enters the blood stream. Other more commonly used "foods" also have a demonstrable, if somewhat less extreme, effect on us. Coffee, for example, stimulates us physically, intellectually, socially, and emotionally, as does sugar. But actually all foods, especially the ones which we eat habitually each day, are affecting each aspect of our being. The effect is less immediate and obvious, but no less profound. Thus, the eggs and bacon I eat for breakfast each day, or the pizza I have for lunch, or the lentil soup and whole-grain bread I take at dinner are also affecting every dimension of my life. They are obviously influencing how my body works, but they are also influencing how I see the world, how I relate to other people, and how I feel about my life.

This view of food as a factor in every aspect of our lives is neither new nor uncommon. From ancient times in many cultures, food has been understood as influencing behavior, personality, values, ideology, and even spiritual life. In India, for example, food has been conceived as dominated by one of three qualities: the pure, calm, harmonious *sattvas*, the active, restless *rajas*, and the diffuse, inactive *tamas*. A person acquires the quality of the food which one eats. A similar understanding of food based on the four cardinal "humors" (the sanguine, choleric, phlegmatic, and melancholic) goes back to Hippocrates and has been present in Western culture since then.

In any case, a basic concept in the Macrobiotic world view is that food is one of the important factors in our life.

6. The optimal diet is ecologically based, consisting of the foods naturally and abundantly present in the immediate environment. In most parts of the world this is a grain-based diet supplemented by other vegetable foods and by small amounts of animal food.

Since food is an important factor in our overall condition, the question of what is proper food is a crucial one. Because the human being is a creature living in nature, we must approach this question by looking at the human being as an eating animal, and by looking at the environment in which he is living.

Sagen Ishizuka (1850–1910) was the Japanese physician who founded the modern Macrobiotic movement, and who was in effect Ohsawa's inspiration and mentor. Ishizuka observed that the human being has the digestive system of a seed and grain eater rather than of a carnivore. Meat-eating animals have sharp teeth for tearing flesh and a large stomach to digest the protein found in meat. The human being has thirty-two teeth, most of which are best suited to chewing seeds and grains. In fact, twenty of our natural teeth are molars, which are like little flour mills, ideal for grinding grains. Also, with its small stomach, and long, convoluted intestines, the human digestive system is best suited to the digestion of complex carbohydrates rather than of proteins.

Ishizuka also observed that in most of the environments where human beings live, the most abundant food crop is one of the cereals. Thus, through history, most major civilizations have had a grain as their principal staple food. In East Asia this was rice and millet; in India, rice and wheat; in Europe, wheat, rye, and oats; in the Americas, maize; and in Africa, millet and sorghum.

He concluded therefore that whole grains should be the principal food of the human being. These should comprise 50 percent or more of the daily food, and should be supplemented by other local foods—beans, vegetables, fruits in season, seeds, nuts, fish and other animal foods. Ishizuka called his dietary philosophy *cerealism*.

Some areas (e.g. far northern Canada) are too cold for grains to grow, however. And some (e.g. the Mongolian steppes) are too dry. Hence Manabu Nishihata, a disciple of Ishizuka, introduced the principle of *shin do fu ji* as the key to the selection of proper food.

This Sino-Japanese phrase has both a literal and a figurative meaning. Literally it means "body and earth not two," or the body and the soil are one. Interpreted more broadly, it means that the human being and the entire natural environment are profoundly related.

The principle is both descriptive and prescriptive. It describes the fact that the human being is a transformation of the natural environment. The atmosphere, the water, the warmth of the sun, and the energy of the earth, directly nourish and sustain us. Transformed into the vegetable kingdom, these elements nourish us indirectly through the plants which we eat for food. Thus we are an ambulatory, talking version of the natural environment in which we live.

Shin do fu ji is prescriptive in that it indicates what foods we must eat to function well and to be healthy in a given environment. It says that we should eat whatever foods grow naturally and abundantly in the area where we live. Nature is a loving and compassionate mother. She provides for all her creatures, including the human being. She provides in the immediate environment those foods most helpful in meeting the demands of that environment. What is growing at our feet and all around us is the ideal food for us.

In most of the regions where human beings live, particularly the temperate zones, cereal grains are indeed the most abundant food crop. So, in such places, the diet should have grains as a principal food, augmented by other local and seasonal foods. Where grains do not grow, the foods that are naturally and readily available are to be eaten. Hence in the arctic, a diet of animal meat, fish, and berries is ecologically appropriate (i.e. Macrobiotic), and in the jungle, one of fruits, tubers, and insects.

There are indeed many factors to be considered in an individual's diet. These include ethnic heritage (especially if the person is living in a place different than that of his forebears), age, sex, amount and type of physical activity, health history, present health, and personal preference. But perhaps the single most important consideration is the immediate environment. We should eat foods which occur naturally and abundantly in our immediate surroundings. That is a first and necessary step to being in harmony with nature, and to establishing our health and happiness.

7. A path to true and total health must include a proper diet, but it must include as well the conscious and insightful cultivation of each area of life, from physical to spiritual.

Certainly food is a crucial factor. But even on the physical level it is only one of many factors. The air we breathe, the kind of clothes we wear, and the exercise we do or do not do are also key elements in our physical and in our general well-being. And each of the other domains of life is equally important. How we nourish and exercise our other bodies—aesthetic, emotional, intellectual, social-moral, ideological, and spiritual—is as important as how we nourish and exercise our physical body. Each is crucial in itself and as a factor affecting all the others.

For example, our emotional well-being requires among other things, self-acceptance, loving and open relationships with family and friends, and a satisfying vocation. Our success in developing these largely determines whether we are happy or unhappy persons. Our emotional condition however, is affecting every other aspect of life. If we are upset about our marriage or job, then our digestion, our ability to see the beauty in the world, our social relations, will all suffer as well.

Thus to rely exclusively on food as a means to achieve health is to invite frustration. It is like driving across the country in a car which has eight cylinders, but only one that works. One will move but with unnecessary slowness and difficulty.

Thus, through food we can initiate and affect changes in our physical body and in each of our other bodies. But the transformation will be faster and more profound if we work on every area directly as well. Energy expended and progress made in one domain of life benefits not just that area, but all the others as well. For example, if I actively cultivate my emotional life (by changing to a more satisfying job, for example), I will become a happier person. My physical condition will directly benefit. And because it is easier for a happy me to follow a wholesome diet, to maintain an exercise program, and do other sensible "healthy" things, my physical health will benefit indirectly as well. The other bodies will also benefit directly and indirectly. In other words, the principle of *synergy* will take effect, and the net result will be greater than the sum of my efforts.

Thus, Macrobiotics as a practical path toward health and happiness includes careful and conscious cultivation of each of the human bodies and of each dimension of life. The following chapters will explore some of the ways we can pursue this.

2. Edible Shampoo, Organic Undershorts, and Other Necessities

> Now I see the secret of making the best persons. It
> is to grow in the open air and to eat and sleep with
> the earth.
>
> Walt Whitman (1819–1892)

The human body resembles an engine. It takes in fuel, burns it to create energy, and gives off waste products. Also, like an engine, it requires air and water to operate. Having the ability to grow, to repair itself, and to reproduce, the body is distinct from an engine, but the similarity does exist.

The smooth (healthy) operation of the human "engine" depends largely on the quality of its fuel. The body's health is much influenced by the food which is eaten and digested. But it is also influenced by the quality of the water and air which are taken in, and by the quality of other, more subtle influences, such as light and electromagnetic energy. There are many books that deal with food and diet from the Macrobiotic viewpoint. And this book expressly is concerned with things other than food. So we will forego a discussion of this primary fuel of the body and consider instead those other forms of nourishment—water, air, light, and energy—which affect our physical condition.

In our modern industrial society we are in a paradoxical situation regarding the necessities for physical health. We are both blessed and cursed. For example, our agricultural and food-processing system has made our food supply plentiful, varied, colorful, convenient, and stimulating to the taste. Unfortunately, most of the foods in our supermarkets, refined, processed, and chemicalized as they are, do not promote our health. To obtain wholesome, life-sustaining food these days requires special effort and attention.

The same is true of the water, air, light, and energy which we require. We are assured of ample, relatively clean (bacteria-free

at least) water. We are assured also of comfortable air—not too
hot, cold, damp, or dry. We have light and energy available to
us at all times. Yet every blessing is a mixed one. We pay a
price for this security, comfort, and convenience. The quality of
what we get is severely compromised. We have water, air, light
and energy but they are of such poor quality that they may not
be able to support our health and well-being.

We human beings are creatures of nature, created and constantly nourished by the elements of the natural world. To be
healthy and happy we need these in their pure, life-giving and
life-sustaining form. So, just as we take trouble to get organic
and unprocessed food, we must take trouble to get good-quality
water, air, light, and energy.

Good Water: Water is the indispensable matrix of life, at
least as we know life on this planet. The human body is over
70 percent water. We are really just large ambulatory sponges.
Were all this water not contained in our cell walls and in our
blood vessels, and were not the whole structure enveloped in
skin and supported by the skeleton, we would be an immense
incontinent amoeba, dripping, squirting, and flopping all over
the place. Quite untidy, indeed. In any case, as the primary
compound in the human body, water obviously plays a key role
in the proper functioning of our biological machine. There is a
proverb in Japanese which states that the "personality" of the
people in a village reflects the quality of the water of the place.

All water is basically the same, each molecule consisting of
two atoms of hydrogen combined with one atom of oxygen.
But in fact waters vary greatly, containing any of a variety of
other substances. These include mineral elements such as calcium, magnesium, iron, and sodium, dissolved organic matter,
living organisms such as bacteria and viruses, as well as human-
made chemicals.

Also, from an energetic viewpoint, water will vary according
to its source and container. Spring water fresh from the ground
has a different energy than the same water that has been sitting
in a bottle for a week. According to the canons of Japanese tea

ceremony, water drawn from the center of a stream is different in quality and taste from that taken from its edge. Rain water which is (or at least, before acid rain, was) relatively pure H_2O, is distinct from the pure water produced by an electric distiller.

What then is ideal water for drinking and cooking? It is water that is free of disease-causing microorganisms, of dissolved organic matter, and of synthetic compounds. If it contains natural minerals, these should be in moderate amounts. Also, it should come directly from nature, from a stream, river, spring, lake, or well, so that it is infused with the vital energy of the earth.

Unfortunately, sources of such water are very scarce and are growing more scarce by the year. All over the planet, in undeveloped nations as well as developed ones, in agricultural and even wilderness areas, as well as urban and industrial regions, good water is increasingly difficult to find. In many places it is impossible to obtain.

Contamination by disease-bearing organisms is common. The same microorganisms that cause dysentery and other gastro-intestinal problems in India and Mexico are present in the mountain streams and lakes of New England. Chemical pollution of the water systems also is widespread. Industrial wastes dumped into water sources or onto the ground, agricultural fertilizers and poisons laid on fields, air pollution brought to the earth by rain, all ultimately find their way into the water system. A friend of mine living in Chicago sent a sample of his tap water to be analyzed and received a sobering report. There were about thirty different petroleum and coal-tar based chemicals in the water, as well as asbestos fibres. Presumably these were present at levels acceptable to the Chicago health authorities, but perhaps not so acceptable to my friend's body and those of his children.

The worldwide water situation today is so grave and deteriorating so rapidly that it is becoming a threat to human survival. While biologically contaminated water is spreading infectious diseases, chemically tainted drinking water is probably contributing to the epidemic of cancer and other systemic diseases.

And since we can live only a few days without water, if our sources ever become totally non-potable, we will soon perish.

Good water then is not only very important, it is like a good man—"very hard to find." What are the possible ways to deal with this situation?

The best solution of course is to have an unsullied stream, well, or spring in your backyard. Such water sources still do exist but they are very rare. The chance of having one close at hand is about the same as winning the state lottery—rather small. Even in many rural areas, water sources, because of agricultural runoff, are polluted. If you do have a local natural water source, be sure to have the water tested. The environmental quality agency in your state will do this or refer you to someone who will. You may be among the lucky few.

Otherwise, start asking around about sources of good water in your area. Ask the people at your natural foods store, ask state park officials, local farmers, even strangers in the street. Keep at this as if your life depended on it. Eventually you will find an accessible source of good water within a reasonable distance of your home. When you do, make sure that it has been tested recently. Then get a number of one-gallon or five-gallon glass bottles and plan to visit this source on a regular basis. One person will use four to five gallons per week of water for drinking and cooking. Avoid plastic bottles since they affect the chemical content, taste, and energy of the water. After a couple of days in a plastic bottle even the best water will be seriously compromised.

One can also buy the bottled water that is sold in most natural foods stores and in many supermarkets. This is very convenient of course. But, even if the water is indeed what it is said to be, namely pure well or spring water, there are disadvantages to it. Probably the water has been sitting in those one gallon-plastic jars for quite a while. Thus it has lost its original energy and is no longer chemically pure. If you must use bottled water, try to get it in glass bottles. Also, before you use it, take off the top and agitate the water in a spiralic or circular way for a minute of two. This may remind the water of its happier past gurgling down a boulder-strewn stream, and may give it a bit more UMPHH. Some people claim that a quartz crystal, left out in the sun or placed in a real live stream, and then put in a bottle of water, also will improve the energy of water.

Another approach is to buy a water distiller. This is an electrical machine which boils and then condenses water, producing more or less pure H_2O. Bacteria are destroyed and minerals and particulate matter are left as a sediment. Many health advocates recommend distilled water saying that it is like rain water and keeps excess minerals out of the body. This is true, but energetically, distilled water—electrically heated and then condensed in metal tubes—is different than the rainwater which falls from the sky. Also, the minerals, if not in excess, give water taste and body and can be a source of nourishment.

One can also invest in a water filter. These devices, attached to the water faucet or to another point in the water system, filter the water as it is used. There are a variety available. Some take out organic pollutants; some remove chemical pollutants as well. Some take out the naturally occurring minerals, some leave them in. If you do decide to buy one, do thorough research and be clear about exactly what you want. Also be prepared to spend a couple of hundred dollars for a good device. A water filter is an excellent investment, especially for people who cannot find good sources of natural water in their area.

For the wilderness camper and for the international traveler (especially to the Third World), care about water is very important. Dysentery, giardia, and hepatitis are all contracted through bad water. There are several approaches to the problem. One is to boil all water for at least twenty minutes. Another is to treat all water with tincture of iodine and let it stand for twenty minutes before drinking. Unfortunately, the resulting water does not taste very good, and taking in iodine for extended periods may cause problems.

Also, one can use a portable filter. The Swiss-made Katadyne filter, for example, is about the size of a flashlight. It pumps water through a silver-impregnated ceramic filter, and removes all pathogens. It is not cheap (at about $175) but neither is coming down with cholera, dysentery, or hepatitis. The company markets a large, also hand-pumped and portable filter for about $450. This device can furnish enough drinking water for a large family in camping or emergency situations.

None of these solutions is ideal. They all violate the archetypal image we hold in our ancestral memory, that of kneeling beside a spring, stream, or lake and drinking the clear, chill water with delight and trust—of taking the crystal milk of Mother Earth directly from her breast. But we do not live in an ideal world and we must do the best we can under the circumstances. Unfortunately, the situation will get worse before it gets better.

At present we are fortunate that sources of pure water still do exist here and there. We are also fortunate that the technology exists to render polluted water into a relatively potable and safe substance. Clean and natural water not only is delicious, it is necessary to our physical health. We should spare no effort or expense in getting the best water possible for our daily use.

Good Air: While we can live several weeks without food, and several days without water, we can live only a few minutes without air. From the moment we are born to the moment we die, we are constantly taking in air in order to live. Air is a gaseous "food" and its quality also affects our health and well-being.

As with water, the basic composition of the atmosphere is universal. It consists of about 78 percent nitrogen and 18 percent oxygen, with the balance including carbon dioxide, hydrogen, helium, and other rare, inert gases. But in fact air varies greatly. In a crowded room the percentage of oxygen will fall and that of carbon dioxide rise. In a thick forest the opposite may be true. The electrical charge of air varies as molecules gain or lose electrons. The atmosphere holds varying amounts of natural substances such as water vapor and dust. It can also hold gases and particulate matter generated by human activity— such as carbon monoxide, sulfuric acid, and lead.

What then is "good air," an atmospheric environment which will allow us to function optimally? Again, our standard is what Mother Nature supplies to us in normal circumstances. This is air that is free of chemical and particulate pollution, and which contains at least 18 percent oxygen. Also, it is electrically charged air, with about 1,000 ions per cubic centimeter, and with five negative ions to every four positive ions. This is the electrical charge of fresh air in a grassy, sunny field, for example, or next to a stream, or waterfall, or on an ocean beach.

Actually, it is often easy to determine the quality of air. It affects our physical energy and mental acuity very quickly and noticeably. If we are in a closed, crowded room, where there is inadequate oxygen, or in a factory where many electrical machines have positively ionized the air, we soon feel lethargic and oppressed. And, if we walk out of doors and into a breezy field, our energy and mood immediately improve. Good air has an immediate beneficial effect on us, and doubtless it has a long-term positive affect on our health as well.

All over the world, wherever there are cars, trucks, and buses, power plants, and industrial facilities, air quality is a problem. The air pollution in Third World cities such as Mexico City and Bangkok is more severe than that of New York and Tokyo. Even in relatively pristine areas one may smell the stench of a paper mill.

How then can we get good air? If we must live in an urban or congested area this is a real challenge. We can use and promote the use of bicycles and public transportation rather than private automobiles, but we cannot immediately change the general situation much. We can however choose to live and work away from major thoroughfares. Pollution levels are highest at street level on busy traffic arteries.

Otherwise we must do our best to make the best of another less than ideal situation. Each day, early in the morning before rush hour, and in the evening when the pollution of the day has been dispersed, the quality of the air, especially in parks and wooded areas, is relatively good. At those times some mild exercise can be very helpful. Take a vigorous walk and perhaps do some deep breathing exercises. Then at least twice a day the lungs and cells will be treated to a feast of oxygen-rich, relatively clean air.

Most of us spend a good part of our time indoors. There we can influence the quality of the air much more. Of course the basic quality of the air in our homes, offices, and factories is first determined by the quality of the outside atmosphere. Yet we can affect it greatly for ill or for good. In a building or room with a ventilation system, for example, an air filter can remove much dust and dirt.

Actually much indoor air pollution comes from the indoor environment itself. Our homes, offices and factories are polluted from within. For example, building materials, such as particle board, may contain formaldehyde and other chemicals which are slowly, constantly released into the internal environment. Other sources at home and at work include items of everyday use: aerosol sprays, (hair nets, perfumes), stains and paints, shoe polish, nail-polish remover, window cleansers, strong soaps, oven cleaners, magic markers, glue, and typewriter correction and copier fluids. Anything that has a strong odor is giving off molecules into the air. And since most of these products are made from petrochemicals or coal-tar derivatives, what they are giving off is probably harmful. Even gas stoves introduce pollutants into the household atmosphere and must be very well ventilated.

In a tightly insulated environment, this type of air pollution can create a serious problem. A home in a rural area may actually be as polluted as one in the middle of New York City. The solution is twofold. Periodically, even in winter, we can ventilate the house regularly and/or always keep one window slightly open. Also, we can cut down on our use of products which pollute the air.

Although we are used to our roll-on shoe polishes, spray paints, and magic markers, most of these products appeared on the market just in the past several decades. Before that there were natural, non-toxic products serving the same purposes. Most of these are still available. Three books which deal with the issue of indoor pollution, give ways to combat it, and list sources of natural alternatives to toxic products are: *Non-Toxic and Natural* by Deborah Lee Dadd (Jeremy Tarcher, L.A. 1984); *The Non-Toxic Home,* also by Dadd and published by Tarcher in 1986; and *Why Your House May Endanger Your Health* by Alfred Zamm (Simon and Schuster, 1980).

The electrical charge of the air is very important. Research indicates that air ionization affects our ability to absorb and to use oxygen. Thus our physical and mental condition is radically affected by the ion balance. An optimal balance helps us feel relaxed, energetic, and optimistic. An unfavorable balance can contribute to lassitude, restlessness, confusion, depression, and even loss of sexual appetite.

Again, we can do little to affect the general atmospheric environment, whose ionization is determined by weather patterns, geography, and levels of air pollution. We can however do much to control the ion situation in our indoor environment.

Certain factors create a beneficial ion balance, by generating negative and by absorbing positive ions. These include fresh air ventilation; sunshine; moving water (as in a fountain); regular dusting and mopping; and furniture, floor coverings, and upholstery made of natural materials such as wood, cotton, and wool. House plants promote a "friendly" ion environment and also enrich the air with oxygen. Plants are our "partners in breath," during the daytime breathing in the carbon dioxide, which we give off as waste, and breathing out the oxygen which we need to live. Thus, having household plants can greatly improve an indoor atmosphere.

Other factors create an unfavorable ion balance. These include forced-air heating systems, air conditioners, electrical motors and appliances (such as heaters, computers, and televisions), dust and dirt, excessively dry air, and furnishings and carpets made from synthetic and plastic materials.

By maximizing the one and minimizing the other we can create a pleasant and healthy indoor environment. This may involve expense and inconvenience. Wooden furniture is more

costly than that made from plastic or steel. It is a burden perhaps to dust, sweep, and mop every day. But the immediate and
long-term benefits are real and worth the effort.

Usually in a book about healthful living one could expect to
dispense with the topic of smoking in a few well-chosen words.
For example, "SMOKING IS AN EXCELLENT METHOD
OF SLOW MOTION SUICIDE," would usually suffice. But
alas, in a book concerning Macrobiotics, such is not the case.

The Macrobiotic movement has always discouraged the use of
recreational drugs. Even in the heyday of the drug culture,
teachers and serious students of Macrobiotics unequivocally
condemned all drugs, including marijuana. Still today, drugs are
understood as extreme and dangerous substances, which may
have an immediate pleasant or beneficial effect, but which in
fact cause great harm. Nicotine, however, has escaped this con-
demnation and cigarette smoking has been in the past, and is
today, practiced and accepted within the Macrobiotic community. To understand this paradox we must look at the early
history of Macrobiotics in the West.

Mr. Ohsawa was a heavy smoker who enjoyed both cigarettes
and pipe tobacco. In the late 1950s and early 1960s, when the
medical community and general public began to realize that
smoking was related to cancer and other illnesses, Ohsawa was
often questioned about his habit. Sometimes he would reply: "I
smoke because I am not an angel." This was an excellent retort
since indeed none of us are angels and all of us harbor some
vice, major or minor, that is self-destructive. However, Ohsawa
decided to take the offense. He began to claim (most noticeably
in *Zen Macrobiotics*), that smoking is not harmful. He claimed
that it could be beneficial, could in fact help cure cancer.

Ohsawa argued that tobacco is a very Yin, expanded plant
which when dried, aged, shredded, and rolled, becomes very
Yang. When this product is burned—further Yangized—it yields
a very Yang influence. Since cancer usually is a condition of
excess Yin, smoking is not the cause. The real cause is excess
Yin food: refined sugar, white flour, excessive amounts of animal
fat, and chemical additives. In fact, if these are eliminated from

the diet, according to Ohsawa, tobacco can be used to cure cancer.

Preposterous as this sounds, there may be some truth in it. Among peoples whose diet is low in fat and refined products, the Andean villagers of Peru for example, smoking does not usually lead to cancer. And some traditional medical systems, including that of the Chinese, use tobacco to treat certain illnesses.

In a broad sense, tobacco is a "food." If it is used according to the principles of quality and quantity (as all foods should be used), then it may indeed be beneficial, or at least not harmful. For example, I could get the best quality, organically-grown tobacco, and smoke it once a day or once a week in order to relax, to focus my mind, or to enrich a social situation. The tobacco will provide some benefits (emotional, mental, social) and probably will not be physically harmful.

As smoking is generally practiced today, however, it is a grievous health hazard, both for those who smoke and those in their company, the "passive smokers." Tobacco, since it is not considered a food crop, is treated heavily with agricultural poisons. Then, in the manufacturing process, many chemicals are used, including saltpeter, formaldehyde, and sugar. Thus most commercial cigarettes are saturated with chemicals. Then, of course, few smokers enjoy one or two cigarettes a day. In fact, addicted to the nicotine in the tobacco, they are more likely to smoke twenty or thirty. This type of smoking seems to work against that realization of physical and mental health which is the aim of Macrobiotics.

Nevertheless there are many Macrobiotic people, including teachers and leaders in the movement, who smoke. Ohsawa's example and justification are behind this to some extent. They make smoking the permissible sin, a form of self-indulgence still available to people who have given up hamburgers, French fries, and chocolate chip ice cream.

In part, smoking may be due to an overly narrow diet and a lack of exercise. According to traditional Chinese medicine, foods can be classified according to the five "elements," or "stages of energy": wood, fire, soil, metal and water. The standard Macrobiotic diet, particularly in its popular Japanese form, consists largely of "metal" energy foods, such as rice, soybeans, daikon radish, and salt. These are very contractive and require for balance "fire" foods, such as corn and peppers, which are seldom used.* Smoking then may result from a desire for the relaxing, ethereal fire energy. It is relevant perhaps that in Japan and China about 75 percent of the adult males smoke.

For a Macrobiotic person who wants to reduce or give up smoking, the following steps may be helpful:

- Reduce consumption of pressure-cooked rice, miso, and other contractive or salty foods.
- Eat a light and broad form of the diet, including lighter grains, noodles, lightly cooked and raw vegetables, sprouts, cooked and raw fruits.
- Develop a program of daily, mild aerobic exercise and/or deep breathing.
- Use only cigarettes, such as Balkan Sobranie's and Sherman's, made from fine, unadulterated tobacco.
- Make smoking into a special and occasional act rather than a habitual one.

Good Light: Light is also in a broad sense "food." It is a form of electromagnetic energy and hence seems distinct from material sources of nourishment such as vegetable and animal products, water and air. But the distinction is more apparent than real. Matter and energy are just forms of one another. Matter is concentrated, slowly moving energy; energy is diffuse and rapidly vibrating matter. Light is a relatively subtle form of nourishment and sustenance but it is as necessary as food, water, or air. We need good quality light to be active and well. Without it we become lethargic and ill.

Much of what is known about the importance of light is the

* Jack Garvey in his excellent book *The Five Phases of Food*, (Well-Being Books, 1985) was the first to call attention to this issue.

result of the work of Dr. John Ott. Twenty-five years ago Ott became interested in the field of *Photo-biology*, the study of the effect of light on living organisms. Conducting his own laboratory research and referring to the work of others, Ott discovered that light plays a crucial role in life processes, and that plants, animals, and human beings respond very differently to different types of light. In his book, *Health and Light*, published first in the early 1970's and currently available from Pocket Books, Ott presents his key findings. It is unfortunate that his work has been little heeded, since its implications for human health are very great.

Not surprisingly, the ideal type of light, according to Ott, is natural light from God's own light bulb—the sun. Sunlight contains a broad range of the electromagnetic spectrum, including ultraviolet to infrared waves, as well as all the visible wave lengths. This "full spectrum" is necessary for the proper functioning of the human organism. Thus, people deprived of sunlight, experience physical and mental lassitude, depression, and anxiety. And conversely, people suffering from such symptoms may gain relief merely from exposure to natural light. Ott hypothesizes that the key is the pineal gland. Located behind the bridge of the nose, between the eyes and the brain, this small gland seems to be related to the functioning of the *pituitary* gland. The pituitary is the master control of the endocrine system and regulates all the metabolic processes of the body. The optic nerves converge at the pineal and pass around and through it. Thus the different types of light falling on the eye and stimulating the optic nerve may affect the activity of the pineal, and in turn the pituitary. Whatever the mechanism, it is clear that natural sunlight is needed for the healthy functioning of body and mind. The "cabin fever" people experience from spending the winter months indoors results in good part from deprivation of natural light.

Natural sunlight is important because of its relation to Vitamin D as well. Vitamin D is necessary for calcium and phosphorus metabolism (particularly in the formation of bones and teeth), to heart action, nervous-system maintenance, and for normal blood clotting and skin respiration. It occurs naturally in fish liver oil, and is usually added in a synthetic form to commercial milk.* However, for a vegetarian or Macrobiotic person not using these foods, the prime source of vitamin D is sunlight. Under the direct stimulation of natural light the human skin is able to synthesize the vitamin. Therefore, for a Macrobiotic person, regular, preferably daily exposure to sunlight (minimally 20 to 30 minutes) is essential. Otherwise, bone problems, such as *osteoporosis*, and other difficulties may result.

In any case, natural sunlight is necessary for human health. Thus it is important that we get outside every day, rain or shine, for at least half-an-hour. It is not necessary that the sun be out. The sun is of course always shining, even on overcast days. And most of the beneficial rays get through the clouds. Conventional sunglasses are not desirable except under very extreme circumstances. These block out some of the very beneficial wave lengths of the spectrum. For the same reason, a person who wears glasses should try to be outdoors without them as much as possible. Special "full spectrum" lenses, both clear and tinted, are available and are claimed to block out very little of the healthful natural-light spectrum.

Of course, one can get too much of a good thing. And there is today concern about the ill affects of exposure to sunlight— including premature aging and skin cancer. Several factors must be considered however. The people most often affected are fair-skinned Caucasians living in or visiting a tropical or subtropical area. Probably, they are spending long periods each day in the sun and are eating a diet rich in animal foods and refined products. The cause of the problem is less the sunlight than the various ways these people are violating, albeit unconsciously, the order of nature.

Firstly, the white races evolved in the northern, temperate

---

* There are two types of vitamin D, called D_2 and D_3. D_3 is the naturally occurring form of the vitamin. D_3 that is added to milk however is usually a synthetic copy of the real thing. D_2 is an artificial analog with a different molecular structure. According to some experts D_2 has serious adverse effects. It should be avoided.

zones where sunlight is relatively scarce and weak. Hence, they have little natural tolerance for strong sunshine. Also, human beings are meant to be active and mobile. We are not meant to lie inert and motionless like a lizard in the blazing sun. A person who does so runs the risk of something, of terminal boredom at the least. Finally, an appropriate diet in a tropical climate should be based on local, natural foods in their whole forms. Thus, a Caucasian person who goes to a hot country, who lies fully exposed in the sun for hours at a time, and who eats an ecologically inappropriate diet, is violating the order of nature in three significant ways. If he protects himself with light clothing, (as many native peoples themselves do), is moderately active, and eats an ecologically appropriate (i.e. Macrobiotic) diet, the danger from the strong sun will be greatly reduced. The same precautions apply to the summer season in a temperate climate. As Noel Coward said, "Only mad dogs and Englishmen go out in the midday sun!"

Most people spend a good part of their lives indoors under some form of artificial light. In the past, candles and lamps fueled with oil or gas provided this indoor illumination. Today various types of electric lights do so. None of these sources are as good as the sun—God's light bulb. Each has its advantages and disadvantages.

There is a certain appeal to candlelight and even to the light of a kerosene lantern. It is soft, mellow, and relaxing. Such light is nostalgic as well, reminding us of a simpler, but now lost way of life. Candles, lanterns, and gas lamps can still be used in situations where a soft, diffuse light is appropriate: an evening meal, a session of listening to music, an intimate conversation. However, they provide a relatively weak and flickering light, and when used on a mass scale they can be inconvenient and dangerous. For these reasons, most of the world has turned to electric lights.

Electric lights are indeed convenient. And they provide bright and constant light. But they are not ideal. Some types in fact are harmful and pose a threat to human health.

The two most common types of electric lights are incandescent and fluorescent. Incandescent bulbs, most of which still have the classic pear shape, contain a tiny coiled wire or filament in a vacuum. When electrical current passes through this wire, the filament gives off light and heat. Incandescent lights are relatively innocuous. They do not generate a full spectrum but they come close enough that most people can function under them with no problem.

Fluorescent lights are long tubes, filled with a gas and coated on the inside with a fluorescent substance. When a stream of electrons passes through the tube, the coating "fluoresces" or gives off light. Fluorescent lights use less electricity than incandescent lights. Also, they give off a very bright and diffuse light. Hence they are to be found in most schoolrooms, offices, factories, and retail stores.

Unfortunately, fluorescent lights have some serious disadvantages. They give off an imbalanced range of visible light waves, and thus radically distort colors. If you look at yourself in the mirror under bright fluorescent lights you may appear a bit yellow and orange, which at the least is not good for the ego. They also lack many of the invisible wave lengths, such as the benefical "near-ultraviolet rays." Because of the alternating nature of electrical current, fluorescent lights flicker at high rates, about sixty times per second. Moreover, they give off a low, but audible hum as well as low levels of ionizing radiation (X-rays) from their cathodes. This all adds up to that fluorescent lights severely stress the human eye and the entire human body.

In his book, Ott cites sobering studies which indicate that fluorescent lights can cause eye strain, restlessness, hyperactivity, inability to concentrate, anxiety, and even serious mental depression. In the same way that natural light affects the human organism in a positive way by stimulating the optic nerve and the pineal and pituitary glands, fluorescent lights seem to negatively affect the whole system.

Another source of inadequate, perhaps dangerous, light is the sodium arc lamp. This is commonly used in street lights, parking lots, and in some school gymnasia. These use very little electricity and give off a distinctive orange light. The ill effects of these lamps are immediate and obvious. In many schools, teachers and students complained of severe eye strain and headaches when under them, and the lamps have had to be replaced. I have seen a dog accompany his mistress to the entrance of a gym brightly illuminated with sodium lights, take one look at them, and refuse to go in. These lights are sometimes called "crime prevention" lights, probably because when muggers lurk under them waiting for prey, they sicken and die within a few hours.

Thus the "light" food which we encounter in our modern environment is often not ideal. In fact, it may be a serious hazard to our health. It is important that we minimize its ill effects. Fortunately we can do this by observing the following suggestions:

- Utilize natural light from windows and skylights as much as possible.
- Use special "full spectrum" eye-glass lenses, sunglasses, and windowpanes. These let through, in addition to all the visible rays, the near-ultraviolet waves which are important to us.
- Use incandescent lights rather than fluorescent or sodium arc lights. If necessary, replace fluorescent lights with incandescent fixtures. Even in an office situation this is not difficult. A fluorescent bulb above one's desk can be easily disengaged and a desk lamp can be used to supply adequate light.
- Use full-spectrum bulbs. There are both full-spectrum incandescent and fluorescent bulbs available. These duplicate, more or less, the wave spectrum of natural light. Because of the hum and flicker of fluorescent lighting, regular incandescent light may be preferable to a full-spectrum fluorescent light. There are, however, "full-spectrum" fluorescent fixtures which have shielded cathodes to eliminate radiation.
- Use only the amount of artificial light that is necessary. Many household rooms, particularly kitchens, as well as

many offices and stores, are vastly over-illuminated. High-wattage incandescent lighting and continuous banks of fluorescent lamps are unnecessary in most situations.

Ch'i (Ki) or Proto-Energy: There is another type of "food" yet more ethereal than visible light but also necessary to our health and well-being. This may be called in a broad sense "electro-magnetic energy," or "proto-energy," or in Chinese terminology, *Ch'i.*

Most traditional cultures have recognized the existence of this invisible, intangible force, which is essential to life. The Japanese call it *Ki*, the Indians *prajna*, the Arabs *baraka*, and the Poly-nesians *mana*. In Western culture it is most commonly called "spirit." The French philosopher Henri Bergson called it *élan vital* ("vital energy"). Christolph von Hufeland, a German doctor who in 1796 wrote a book called *Macrobiotics, the Art of Prolonging Human Life* (and from whom Ohsawa borrowed the term "Macrobiotics"), called this primal energy *Lebenskraft* or "life force."

From ancient times the Chinese have studied this energetic dimension of reality with particular assiduity. According to the traditional Chinese world view, Ch'i is the primal energy of the universe. It is omnipresent, existing in the air and in the earth and in every particular phenomenon—in each rock, tree, insect, bird, animal, and human being. Within the human body it gives movement and life to the organism.

Ch'i is dynamic, constantly moving, constantly circulating. In relation to the human body there are two primary patterns of circulation. One is internal. Ch'i flows along specific linear pathways or *meridians*, just under the skin of the arms, legs, trunk, and head. The meridians direct the Ch'i around the body and also through the various internal organs. For the proper functioning of the organs and of the body as a whole, there must be a strong and balanced flow of Ch'i throughout the meridian system.

There is also a circulation of Ch'i between the body and the external environment. Particularly at the 365 key points on the

meridians, "tired" Ch'i is being given off by the body and
"fresh" Ch'i is being absorbed from the environment. Most of
this exchange is between the body and the atmosphere, but on
the bottoms of the feet it is between the body and the earth.
This continuous absorption and discharge of Ch'i also is necessary to the proper functioning of the body.

The free flow of energy within the body, and between the body
and the environment, is necessary to our health. Our clothing,
shoes, and jewelry, even our homes and places of work, affect
this circulation of Ch'i. Thus our decisions on what we wear and
where we spend our time can profoundly affect our health and
well-being.

For example, our clothing affects both patterns of Ch'i circulation. Somewhat loose-fitting clothes made of natural fabrics
such as cotton, linen, or wool, are ideal. These impede minimally
the flow of Ch'i through the body and between the body and the
outside environment. Tight-fitting clothes and clothes made of
synthetic materials can have a negative effect. Tight clothes
cause the muscles to tense slightly, reducing circulation of blood
as well as of Ch'i. (Tight pants are especially bad since they also
raise the temperature of the lower abdomen and crotch. These
areas, which are prone to fungus and other infections, should be
kept cool.) Synthetic fabrics disrupt the flow or Ch'i within the
body and also prevent the free circulation of energy between the
body and the air. They are particularly harmful if worn directly
on the skin.

Thus, underwear and clothing of nylon, polyester, and other
synthetics can reduce our physical and mental energy. They can
even affect the proper functioning of our internal organs. It is
not unusual for people who begin eating a Macrobiotic or
natural-foods diet to soon become sensitive to the ill effects of
synthetic clothing. They feel uncomfortable in them and intuitively prefer natural-fibre clothing.

Fortunately, there is an increasing amount of good-quality,
cotton, wool, and even linen clothing available. While definitely
preferable to synthetic items, it is unfortunately still not ideal.
Cotton, for example, is not considered a food crop. Therefore

particularly large amounts of pesticides and herbicides are used in its cultivation. Also, its processing involves many harsh chemicals. And it is usually colored with dyes whose base is *aniline* or *benzidine*, both synthetic chemicals. Thus even a 100 percent cotton pair of pants has a chemical "aura." And if it is an "easy-care" item, it has a chemical finish to prevent wrinkling.

These natural-fibre products are certainly acceptable for the moment. But we should aspire perhaps to a purer quality. A shirt, for example, can be made from cotton that has been organically grown, processed without chemicals, left untreated and then dyed using natural, mineral or vegetable colors. Such a shirt would be a big improvement over the typical all-cotton item of today. And it might have a positive effect on our energy and overall health.

Such products are available, if not easy to find. Traditional woolen clothing—suits, dresses, sweaters, coats—is often "natural" or close to it. And natural clothing in cotton is becoming more available, imported from Third World countries such as India and Guatemala, but also manufactured in Europe and North America. However, these tend to be very casual in style, featuring baggy pull-over shirts and draw-string pants. They mark one as an antiquated Hippie or as a person who has forgotten to take off his pajamas. It is possible though to make stylish, attractive clothing from unprocessed, naturally dyed cotton, linen, wool and silk. Up to a century ago all clothing was natural.

Certainly, there is a market niche here for some enterprising spirit. Someday soon someone will get rich making "organic" clothing that is appropriate for a church service or business meeting as well as for a Yoga class. If it is you, please remember where you got the idea.

The Ch'i of the earth is also necessary to health. This Ch'i is different from that in the atmosphere, being relatively Yin, or cooling, calming, and pacifying. Instinctively, we enjoy touching the earth—by sitting in the grass or walking barefoot on the beach. Unfortunately, today even touching our Mother Earth is very difficult. Much of the ground is covered with asphalt and concrete. Also, our shoes generally are soled with synthetic nonconducting materials, such as synthetic rubber, Vibram, or foam, and these, like synthetic fabrics, act as an insulator. They prevent the free exchange of energy between our bodies and the earth. In a real and substantial sense, they keep us from being "grounded."

Contact with the earth is important to our health. It is important enough that Mr. Kushi in his "general health recommendations," includes walking barefoot in the grass for thirty minutes every morning. This is when the energy of the earth is rising and strong. We can also overcome this insulation and separation from the earth's energy by wearing shoes and socks of natural materials. The shoe's sole is particularly important and should be made of leather or some other natural material. Wooden clogs are available, as are rope-soled sandals, though you have to travel to Central America for the latter. Some very good dress shoes, especially men's, still have leather soles. But in general, the options in buying natural footwear are very limited. Here too, there is a market niche open and waiting for the enterprising, Macrobiotically-oriented entrepreneur. Again we humbly await your generous remembrance.

Jewelry of course can also affect the energy flow in our body. Certain stones and metals, because of their particular qualities, may actually improve it. In fact, the custom of wearing gold, silver, diamonds, crystals, and other precious and semiprecious metals and stones may have originated in part from the recognition that they positively affect physical and mental energy. The specifics of this issue, of course, comprise a vast and complex study in itself. Here, suffice it to say that wearing a piece of jewelry is an important act, and should involve careful study and consideration. At the least, one should wear a new piece for a while and observe what, if any changes it causes. If it proves uncomfortable in one place, try another. A ring worn on one finger may have a different effect when worn on another. And ornaments of plastic and other synthetic materials are probably best avoided entirely. Costume jewelry, while it may look pretty, vibrationally may be the "junk food" of the ornamental world.

We human beings wear clothing, in part from modesty, but primarily to shelter ourselves from the elements. We are actually rather fragile creatures, "naked apes," bereft of substantial protective covering. In our natural state we are able to survive only in a fairly moderate climate where the temperature is comfortable (about 70 degrees Fahrenheit). If the temperature is much lower, or if there is rain and wind, we have difficulty maintaining our normal body temperature. And if the temperature is much above 100°F., and/or the sun is direct upon us, we can become too hot to continue functioning. Thus, in most situations, we need protection from the environment. And the clothing we wear is the first line of defense.

The buildings we erect and live in serve the same basic function. They keep us warm and dry or cool and refreshed, as necessary. In effect, they are stationary suits of clothing, tailored very large to allow us to move around inside them. But while buildings insulate and protect us from the vagaries of the natural environment, it is important that they, as well as our clothing, do not insulate us from the life-sustaining Ch'i in the atmosphere and in the earth.

Ideally, our buildings, like our clothing, should be "loose-fitting" and made of natural materials. In this case, "loose-fitting" means able to be naturally ventilated. Many new buildings, particularly hotels and office buildings are hermetically sealed from the outside world. The windows cannot be opened and all air enters through a ventilation system. It comes in positively ionized (having passed through electrical fans and metal ducts), and with very little Ch'i. In terms of energy, it is "dead air."

Our buildings should also be made of natural materials so that the Ch'i of the atmosphere and the Ch'i of the earth can enter unimpeded. Until recently, all buildings were built of necessity from the natural materials available in a given area. They were set on foundations of stone, brick, or wood, or directly upon the earth. And they were built of stone, brick, wood, reeds, and the like.

Most buildings today are built on a foundation of concrete. This consists of natural materials (sand, gravel, and cement—

made from clay and powdered lime). But these ingredients have been crushed and homogenized and deprived of their natural energy-transmitting structure. A building set on such a foundation is partially cut off from the earth's Ch'i. Then the building itself, and its floors and ceilings, are made of concrete, steel, chemically-treated wood, plastic, and other synthetic materials. Foam and fiberglass are used as insulation. Chemically based stains and paints are used on exterior and interior surfaces. Synthetic carpets and hermetically sealed windows are thrown in for good measure. These various synthetic materials of course impede the flow of Ch'i in and out of the building. The result is an interior environment in which the circulation of Ch'i is inhibited, distorted, and perhaps cut off entirely.

Ideally then, our homes and other buildings should be set on foundations of natural stone, and built of untreated wood and/or natural stone. They should be insulated with natural materials (cotton batting perhaps, or with the corn cobs our forefathers used!). And they should be painted and stained with products derived from natural sources rather than petroleum and coal tar.

For most people, of course, it is hard enough to find or build a place to live in without worrying that it is "organic and natural." However, if we do have the opportunity to build our own shelter, it is not so difficult to make it a natural and healthy one. After all, until a few decades ago, all buildings were constructed in this manner. The necessary materials, including untreated lumber, and paints and stains made from natural sources rather than petroleum, are available. There are companies in Europe and North America which specialize in the manufacture and sale of natural building supplies. Admittedly, to build a natural home today involves extra expense and inconvenience, but it is worth the trouble. Most of us spend about half our lives within our home, eating, sleeping, relaxing. The quality of our lives is certainly affected by the quality of this stationary "suit of clothes."

Thus, in our modern environment, we are often deprived of the primal energy of the earth and atmosphere. However, we are exposed to many human-made electromagnetic influences. These can upset the Ch'i flow of the body. They can also affect the flow of regular electricity in the body. Modern science has discovered that the human body is "electric." Electrical current is constantly circulating in the body. Both the central nervous system and the autonomic nervous system receive and transmit impulses by means of electrical energy. This flow of electricity in the body, necessary to its proper functioning, can be affected by external electromagnetic fields. Every movement of electricity produces such a field. Thus, to maintain the proper flow of Ch'i and of electricity in the body, we must be very careful about all sources of electricity and electromagnetic vibration.

Some specific research has been done on this problem, with disquieting results. One study indicates that vegetation under high-tension power lines is profoundly and negatively affected. Trees, grass, and other plants demonstrate erratic and stunted growth patterns compared with plants even a short distance away from the lines. Another very recent study indicates that people living near power lines have higher than average rates of cancer. Of course, the electrical energy in our homes and offices is much weaker, but we are surrounded by it twenty-four hours a day.

Some people are already acutely aware of this factor. Architects and builders influenced by the work of Rudolph Steiner take into consideration the possible ill effects of electrical fields. In their homes and other buildings they try not to enclose a room with electrical wiring. One of the walls is left without wiring so that a closed electrical "net" is avoided, and so that the energy of the outside natural environment can come in. Such measures are uncommon today, but when we become more aware of the effects of electricity on human health, they may become standard practice. For the health-conscious Macrobiotic person, they are worthy of serious consideration.

A number of the sources of electromagnetic influence are such an integral part of our environment that we take them for granted. For example, many people wear a quartz watch. These are so popular today that it is very difficult to get a mechanically driven timepiece. The quartz watch is a marvelous invention. It contains a small electric battery and a sliver of quartz crystal which can transform electrical energy into mechanical movement. The crystal takes the electric current of the battery and vibrates at a very high, to us almost inconceivable rate, perhaps 140,000 times per second. This vibration, plus the electrical impulse of the battery, creates a small, but actual energy field around the watch. The field is invisible and subtle, but real and able to affect other electromagnetic phenomena.

The wrist, according to traditional Chinese medicine, is an important part of the human anatomy. It has twelve radial pulses, each connected to one of the major organs. Also, six meridians related to such important organs as the intestines, heart, and lungs, pass through the wrist. Thus a watch worn on the wrist and possessing its own energy field may very well affect the body and its energy flow in a significant way. A quartz timepiece is best carried in a handbag, day pack, or attaché case, rather than on the body.

The electrically powered quartz watch is a relatively weak source of electromagnetic influence. We are surrounded by much more powerful ones. Some general rules regarding these nearly ubiquitous influences include the following:

- Avoid or minimize the use of electrical appliances such as electrical heaters and heating systems, air conditioners, electric ranges, and blankets;
- Turn off all appliances when they are not in use;
- Do not keep continuously operating appliances, such as electric clocks, next to beds, desks, and other places where much time is spent.

To live in an un-electrified environment would probably be ideal. In modern circumstances, of course, this is impossible. But one can do things to approach this situation. A company in West Germany is marketing a device which shuts off the electrical current to any room unless an appliance is actually in use. Installed in a bedroom, this device would allow one to sleep in a non-electric situation, which is very restful and pleasant. Once,

on the coast of Maine, I lived in a cabin whose electrical supply
was controlled by an easily accessible switch. Each night before
going to bed I shut the electricity off. The lights went out and
the refrigerator (sparsely stocked and ice-less) stopped, and
a palpable, almost other-wordly silence and calm settled on the
house (and on me).

Actually, there is a much more dangerous vibrational influence
present in our environment, indeed present almost everywhere.
This is radiation. There are two types of radiation. Ionizing
radiation such as that given off by an X-ray machine, causes
molecular change in the body cells. Non-ionizing radiation, such
as that from a television or microwave oven affects the body's
functioning but without creating electrically charged molecules
or ions. Both types of radiation are harmful to the human
organism. We tend to think of radiation as a problem distant in
space and in time, which will affect us in the event of nuclear
war or a major accident at a nuclear power plant. Of course,
since Chernobyl, people in Europe have not had this luxury.

But in fact radiation is a problem here and now. Many,
perhaps most people in modern society are exposed daily to
radiation in their homes and places of work. Few are aware of
this and few are aware that they may be suffering serious negative effects, both short term and long term.

Many of the sources of radiation are so integral to our lives
that we take them for granted and cannot conceive that they
might be harmful. For example, the cathodes of fluorescent
lights, if not properly shielded, give off some radiation. Some
types of smoke alarms operate using radioactive materials, and
microwave ovens also generate ionizing radiation. Admittedly,
the amounts of radiation given off are very small. But despite
the assurances of government and industry, many scientists say
that any amount is unsafe and unacceptable. Such devices have
not been around long enough for their real impact to be studied
or known. Our bodies may undergo changes even with very low
levels of radiation.

Even something as apparently innocuous as a radiant watch
dial is giving off ionizing radiation, which may affect our physical

health. At a lecture in Holland once I mentioned that most radiant dials contain radioactive materials. A gentleman in the first row, who had been battling a malignancy for several years, looked down at his wrist watch in surprise and consternation. "This watch has a radiant dial," he exclaimed, "and I have been wearing it for five years!" Now, in reality, his watch may not have had anything to do with his condition. But it may have. The functioning and malfunctioning of the human body are still in large part mysteries.

The color television and the computer monitor, two familiar features of modern life, are both sources of radiation. Both are based on the same device, the cathode ray tube or CRT. Operating at a very high voltage, this tube sends out a stream of electrons toward the back of the television or monitor screen. The electrons cause certain points on the screen to light up and thus produce an image. Most of the stream of electrons is absorbed but some does escape. Thus, a person watching television or sitting in front of a CRT computer monitor probably is subjected to some level of ionizing radiation. Recent advances in technology have greatly reduced the amount of radiation generated and leaking from color televisions and monitors. But even small amounts may be harmful.

The short-term ill effects of exposure to CRT's are well documented. Even back in the 1960s, doctors and scientists had identified "television syndrome," a combination of lassitude, restlessness, anxiety, sleeplessness, and loss of memory which occurred in children watching television for three or more hours a day. And one need only watch others watching television to observe these effects first hand. There is a slack-mouthed, glassy stare (not caused by the subject matter of the program alone) that afflicts the serious watcher and which indicates a real physical and mental impact. Have you ever had a brilliant idea watching television? It is unlikely, since the energy field of body and mind are so severely affected.

And computer monitors have a similar effect. Even in the short time they have been in use they have been recognized as very hazardous. Headaches, eyestrain, nervousness, menstrual irregularities, and higher than normal rates of miscarriage can afflict the regular user. In some European countries, labor laws restrict the number of hours a day a person can work at a computer monitor.

The long-term implications of regular exposure to television and computer monitors are even more sobering. In *Health and Light*, John Ott describes an experiment he did with a color television. He covered half the screen with radiation-absorbing lead, and the other half with black paper. He then placed a rat in a cage in front of each half, and observed their development and behavior. While the rat in the lead-shielded cage developed normally, the other animal was stunted in its growth, and listless and erratic in its behavior. When asked to recommend a safe viewing distance for watching TV, Ott declined to answer. He had observed negative effects on animals who were fifteen feet away from a color television with two walls in between. Admittedly, the improved color televisions of today emit much less radiation, but there is still cause for concern.

The issue of television watching and of computer use is a serious and complicated one. Television provides a continuous and varied parade of entertainment, some of which is well worth watching. Computers simplify and expedite many tasks. But here as elsewhere in life, there is no "free lunch." For every benefit of most modern technology, there is some negative impact as well. Whatever has a front has a back. Where there is Yin there is also Yang. We can, however, by judicious use, minimize the ill effects.

Possible measures include the following:

- Watch these devices from a distance and at an angle. This is easier of course with a television. Some computers have a detachable keyboard which allows the operator to be several feet distant. Even this is helpful though, since the amount of radiation is reduced to one-fourth if the distance is doubled.
- Limit television viewing and computer use.
- Turn off televisions and computer monitors when they are

not actually being watched, since as long as they are on they are generating radiation.

- Use a black-and-white TV or monitor (which has only one cathode ray tube) rather than a color device (which has three). Replace older models with new, presumably improved ones.
- Use a radiation shield (a lead-impregnated screen) over the computer screen.
- Use a non-CRT computer display. Two new types of screens, not based on the cathode ray tube, are now available. The LCD (Liquid Crystal Display) and the gas-phosphor screens both are flat screens and are used primarily in portable computers. They do not produce radiation. Flat television screens, also without CRTs, are being developed.

Thus, in addition to being nourished and affected by its food (in the narrow sense), the human body is affected by a variety of other foods (in the broad sense): water, air, electromagnetic energy, Ch'i, and radiation. And just as we should use discretion and care in choosing our edible food, we should exercise discretion and care in regard to these other sources of nourishment. It is as critical to our physical and general health to get good water, air, to wear natural clothes, and to avoid disruptive energy sources as it is to eat a sound, wholesome diet every day.

Physical Exercise: Our physical condition is affected not only by what we take in but also by how we use what we take in. This brings us to the crucial issue of exercise.

We human beings evolved over millennia as hunters, food-gatherers, herders, and cultivators. In order to get enough to eat and to survive, we had to be physically active. Thus, the human body developed as a biological machine capable of strenuous and sustained labor.

Movement and exercise are in fact necessary to the health of the organism. When the body is not active it suffers. This fact was recognized as far back as the time of Hippocrates (6th century B.C.). The "Father of Western Medicine" observed that physically inactive people were much more prone to disease. And today, modern medicine has established that sedentary people are much more likely to experience loss of muscle tone, decreased heart and lung capacity, loss of flexibility in joints, high blood pressure, hardening of the arteries, diabetes, anxiety, and depression.

For most of human history, physical inactivity has not been a major problem. More people have suffered perhaps from an excess of work rather than a lack of it. Even with the spread of agricultural civilization, most people had to labor long and hard in order to survive. Women and men dug in the fields, harvested crops, chopped wood, hauled water, and moved themselves and their goods with few or no mechanical aids. Until quite recently only a small privileged minority did not have to work hard physically every day. And these leisure classes kept quite active through hunting, sport, martial practice, and recreational walks. The landed gentry of England as described in the novels of Jane Austen, for example, went on long daily rambles over hill and dale, in foul weather or in fair.

Today, the situation for most people, at least in the developed nations, is quite different. In our "culture of convenience," machines have eliminated much of the labor of daily life. Indoor plumbing and heating, the automobile, tractor, telephone, power lawn mower, the elevator, the Cuisinart food psocessor, and countless other mechanical slaves, do most of our physical work. At home or on the job, few people have to exert themselves physically at all. The homemaker throws the laundry into the automatic washer and sits down in front of the TV. The working spouse sits at a desk, shuffles papers, and talks on the telephone. The typical American expends on a typical day only slightly more energy than if he had stayed in bed.

The unfortunate result is that many people miss the benefits, physical and mental, immediate and long term, which regular physical activity provides. When we are physically active substantial changes occur in the body. Waste products are removed from the cells and fresh oxygen is brought in at a rapid rate. Glycogen stored in the liver is released as glucose into the blood stream. This is delivered along with fresh supplies of oxygen to all the cells, including those of the brain and muscles. Thus, after even light exercise, we feel physically and mentally refreshed.

If we exercise enough to double our pulse and respiration rate, more dramatic changes occur. With such strenuous exercise, the brain produces a type of *neurotransmitter* known as *endorphines*. Neurotransmitters are hormones which establish reactions between brain cells and thus cause certain moods and sensations. The endorphines produced during exercise are chemically similar to morphine, and induce a physical and mental calm, even euphoria. Thus, for several hours after strenuous physical activity, one experiences "runner's high." We and the world seem fresh, clean, and alive. In effect then, each of us has dwelling within us a friendly, benevolent "drug pusher," who for the price of a little perspiration will give a natural, legal, and safe "high."

The long-term benefits of exercise also are varied and profound. They include improvement in the following areas:

- heart and lung efficiency and capacity,
- muscle tone,
- strength and flexibility of tendons, ligaments and joints,
- bone strength (exercise helps bones absorb calcium),
- pulse rate and blood pressure,
- body weight (exercise moderates appetite and burns off fat),
- glucose tolerance (exercise helps the body maintain stable blood sugar levels),
- ability to deal with stress and anxiety,
- level of physical and mental energy,
- memory, self-image and sense of personal efficacy, and last but not least,
- level of sexual hormones.

Thus the physically active person can expect to be more

energetic and cheerful, better-looking, more relaxed and even-tempered, even smarter and sexier than if he didn't exercise. And he is less likely to suffer from both acute and chronic illnesses, including heart disease, diabetes, and arthritis. Conversely, a person who is completely sedentary is deprived of these benefits and is more likely to develop some serious physical problem. Obviously then, it is important that every person be physically active on a regular basis. It is an intrinsic part of human life and necessary to health and well-being.

This does not mean that one has to follow a rigorous and exhausting exercise plan involving running or weight lifting. One can get enough exercise in fairly mild activities and even in doing things that are not specifically "exercise."

There are actually two broad types of exercise. One is *extrinsic* or specific exercise. This involves an activity which is outside our normal daily tasks and is an end in itself. The games and sports we play and the "fitness" activities we engage in are forms of extrinsic exercise.

But there is also *intrinsic* exercise which is part of our normal daily life. This includes walking to the store, gardening, mowing the lawn, and doing the laundry. Today, most of these forms of intrinsic exercise have been made unnecessary by machines. We drive to the store, use a power mower and an automatic washing machine. But we are free to do these daily tasks so that they do provide exercise. We can walk or cycle rather than drive; we can use a push mower; we can walk to our seventh-floor office rather than take the elevator. In a great variety of ways we can use our bodies rather than machines in the course of daily life. And in the process, not only will we get some exercise, we will spare the environment some noise and pollution.

Most types of intrinsic exercise, however, are rather mild. They usually do not produce the elevated pulse and respiration rate which are associated with the more profound benefits of exercise. Also, they tend to be relatively inefficient. A busy person may be loathe to spend time washing his clothes by hand, or cycling twenty miles to work. Hence, some kind of regular extrinsic exercise is helpful, even necessary.

The healthy human body possesses five principal characteristics. An ideal program of extrinsic exercise should develop each of these physical attributes. They include:

- Cardiovascular strength, i.e. the ability of the heart, lungs, and circulatory system to deliver oxygenated blood to the body's cells and to remove wastes. This capacity is perhaps the single most important factor in physical fitness.
- Muscle strength and tone.
- Eye-hand and eye-foot coordination.
- Muscle flexibility.
- Strong and balanced Ch'i flow.

Aerobic exercise is exercise that, by strengthening the heart and lungs, increases the efficiency of the body in absorbing oxygen. It usually involves the gross and fairly rapid movement of the limbs and body for twenty minutes or more. Walking, jogging, running, swimming, bicycling, rowing, and "Aerobics" are all forms of aerobic exercise. They strengthen the cardiovascular and respiratory systems, and usually strengthen and tone the muscles as well. Thus, regular, preferably daily, aerobic exercise is a necessary base for a sound fitness program.

Probably the simplest, safest, most convenient, and most generally beneficial, exercise is walking. It can be enjoyed with cardiovascular and muscular benefit by almost anyone regardless of their age or condition. It requires no special equipment, except a pair of good, sturdy walking shoes. It can be done alone or in the company of friends or pets. It gets us out into the fresh air and sunshine. And it does not involve the physical stress and danger of injury associated with running. As a form of exercise however, walking must be distinguished from strolling. It is a vigorous activity, which includes long, fairly rapid strides and a vigorous movement of the arms.

"Race walking," also known as "striding" is an even more rigorous form of exercise. It requires that one's heel strike the ground first and that the leg be straightened with each stride. The resulting swivel-hipped, unusual motion may attract unwanted attention but it promotes flexibility.

Swimming is also an excellent aerobic exercise. It uses many muscles of the body, maintains flexibility, and involves virtually no danger of injury. Swimming in a lake or in the ocean is of course preferable to swimming in a chlorinated pool where one absorbs the toxic chlorine through the skin and inhales it through the lungs.

For each person, because of individual body type, physical condition, and personality, there is an exercise which is most suitable. It should be something one enjoys, which can easily be incorporated into one's daily routine, and which will not be stressful mentally or physically.

Most of the popular sports, such as basketball, volleyball, baseball, tennis, soccer, and racquetball, develop cardiovascular efficiency and muscle tone. They also develop eye-hand coordination. This is very important since it strengthens and stimulates the nervous system. Ping-pong and juggling accomplish the same end.

Coordination between the eyes and feet is also important. If the lower extremities are made "smart," another substantial part of the nervous system is developed. Soccer develops this, as does dance. Recently, a sport called "hackeysack" has become popular. It is an American Indian game in which players stand in a circle and keep a small, soft ball aloft using only their legs and feet. For Americans, accustomed mainly to eye-hand sports, learning to use one's feet well is an interesting and broadening experience.

Muscle flexibility is also very important to physical condition. Flexibility involves the suppleness of the muscles, tendons, and ligaments of the body, particularly those which support the spine. This flexibility is a crucial factor in our general health. The process of aging is largely a process of stiffening, of the gradual loss of flexibility. Infants, whose arms and legs are almost rubbery, are very flexible, as are small children. As we pass through adolescence and then into adulthood this flexibility disappears. Old people tend to be quite stiff. To some degree, this loss of flexibility may be inevitable. But today it is occurring with unnecessary quickness.

This early loss of suppleness is in part due to diet, particularly to excessive amounts of animal fat and animal protein. In part, it is due to the unnatural and stressful body positions which modern life requires of us. Sitting in a car seat or at a desk for hours, or standing all day on a hard floor, perhaps while repeating the same hand motions hundreds of times (as on an assembly line), stresses the body. It creates tension and imbalance in the muscles which can lead to problems in the spine and joints. Rigorous aerobic exercise, such as bicycling or running (especially when done to excess), can also lead to muscle tension. Repeated, rapid movements tighten and shorten muscles. Thus, some kind of flexibility exercise is very important.

Western calisthenics, stretching exercises, and gymnastics, as well as many forms of dance, all aim at the maintenance of flexibility. These are all excellent. The techniques of *Hatha Yoga*, imported from India, are also very good. Hatha or physical Yoga is an ancient and highly developed system for maintaining flexibility and balance of the entire body. It stretches and tones the muscles and other soft tissues. It keeps the joints limber and the spine straight and flexible. Yoga *asanas* or poses are easy to learn, and a fifteen- or twenty-minute session can help keep the body quite flexible. Yoga must be done properly to be truly beneficial. Instruction from a qualified instructor is recommended. Fortunately, classes are given in most parts of the country. Yoga, which also includes breathing and meditational exercises, benefits the mind as well as body.

Exercises designed to strengthen and balance Ch'i flow are also important. The proper circulation of Ch'i is crucial to the harmonious functioning of the whole body. The health of the muscles, soft tissues, the skeleton, and of the internal organs, are all profoundly affected by it. The Japanese martial arts, such as Aikido, Judo, and Karate, and the Chinese exercise systems such as T'ai Ch'i and Ch'i Kung, all benefit Ch'i flow. Perhaps the most convenient form of Ch'i-oriented exercise is *Do-In* (pronounced "dough-een"). This is a form of self-massage in which important acupuncture points are stimulated to improve Ch'i flow. It is easily learned from books (there are several good ones available), and if practiced for a half hour can stimulate energy and create a sense of well-being.

Since no single form of exercise develops all the attributes of the healthy body, an ideal fitness program will include two or more activities. But it need not be complicated or time consuming. An adequate regime might include, for example, a rigorous twenty minute walk each day, followed by another twenty minutes of stretching and Do-In. Most of us fritter away that amount of time each day watching frivolity on television, or catching up on the latest catastrophes in the newspaper. An ambitious program might include as well a few minutes of juggling (for eye-hand coordination) plus a little time kicking around a soccer ball (for eye-foot coordination).

One important consideration in all physical activity, intrinsic and extrinsic, is balance. It is important that the muscles, joints, and tendons and ligaments of both sides of our body develop equally. Otherwise various problems may arise. Therefore we should use and develop both sides of our bodies equally.

Most people in the various activities of daily life, in dressing, cooking, eating, and driving, and in athletic activities, tend to favor one side over the other. A right-handed person, for example, will use his right hand whenever dexterity or strength is required. He will leave his left hand idle or employ it only in a helping role. As a result, the muscles of the right hand, arm, and shoulder, become larger and stronger than those of the left side. This creates a condition of imbalance throughout the muscular and skeletal system. One shoulder may be more tense, and held higher, may cause the hips to be uneven. Imbalance in the muscles of the shoulders and back may cause the vertebrae of the spine to be out of alignment. This will adversely affect the flow of neural stimulation to the internal organs. Also, if we use one hand and arm more than the other, there is unequal stimulation of the Ch'i meridians, and thus of the internal organs. Favoring one hand over the other therefore can have far-reaching negative effects.

To help develop "even-sidedness" one can follow the "Tao of Ambidexterity," known more mundanely as "the two-handed program." This approach develops the strength and dexterity of our "weaker" hand, so that there is more or less parity with the dominant one. I, for example, am right-handed and ordinarily do everything, from brushing my teeth to opening the car door, with that dominant hand. Since beginning the Tao of Ambidexterity, I have used my left hand a great deal more. Thus, in one-handed operations such as eating, shaving, and opening doors, I use it rather than the right. And in two-handed operations such as scrubbing the floor and washing dishes, I use it as the dominant one, and the right hand as the helper. The effect of such a program is noticeable and interesting. Very quickly the long-neglected hand gains in strength, dexterity, and confidence. And each time it masters a new task one feels a thrill of accomplishment, much like that experienced at age five when one learned to tie one's shoes.

The Tao of Ambidexterity is simply an application, a minor one perhaps, of the principle of balance, of Yin and Yang. But it can contribute to that state of harmony and balance, physical and not physical, which we call health. Its implications may be very great. If through the practice of the Tao of Ambidexterity, a person can balance the right and left sides of his body, then all phases of his life may become more balanced and harmonious. He may become thereby a happy and peaceful individual. And as Confucius points out, happy and healthy individuals are the necessary building blocks for a peaceful society. Ambidextrous, happy individuals will create, in turn, peaceful families, communities, nations, and perhaps even a peaceful world. What humanity needs perhaps, is a "World Peace Through Ambidexterity" movement, the international sign of greeting for which is the two-handed handshake.

Body Care and Hygiene: Like any machine or organism involved in the transformation of energy, the human body produces waste materials. Most is excreted as feces and urine. Much however is discharged through the skin, the largest organ of the body and a major organ of excretion. On the skin, body oils and the residue of perspiration mix with dust and dirt from the ex-

ternal environment. The pores of the skin can become clogged,
thus hindering efficient elimination. Also, Ch'i flow along the
skin and through the internal organs can be disrupted. Thus,
proper body hygiene is important to our general physical health.

Macrobiotic people, particularly those who abstain from animal
products and from oily and rich foods, soon discover that diet
affects the amount and quality of the substances which come to
the skin's surface. One's hair and skin become less oily. Underarm odor lessens and even disappears. One's toilet kit can be
reduced to a minimum: a mild facial and body soap, a shampoo,
and a toothbrush and toothpaste.

In choosing these items and any other body-care products
(body lotion, facial cream, hair rinse, lipstick, cosmetics), it is
important to keep one fact in mind. Whatever we put on our
skin finds its way into our bloodstream. The skin seems like
an impermeable shield which protects us totally from the environment. Actually it is highly permeable and whatever comes
in contact with it is absorbed to some degree. Thus, we should
be as careful about what we use on our body as about what
we put in our mouths. Whatever we put on our skin just for
a few moments—soap, toothpaste, shampoo—or for a longer
period—moisturizer, face and hand cream, deodorant, make-up—
should be made of natural, nontoxic ingredients. Thus, our body-
care products should contain only minimally processed vegetable,
animal, or mineral products, and no synthetic substances derived
from coal tar or petroleum.

There are today a number of companies producing, with
varying degrees of strictness, natural toiletries. You will see their
products in your natural foods store. Even there, however, it is
wise to read the label carefully. Some natural products contain
synthetic substances. And many are made primarily with chemical substances derived from plants, which can be as problematic
as petroleum derivatives. I look for products with a few, simple,
familiar ingredients.

We should also be careful with other household products
which come in contact with the skin. Thus dish-washing soap
should be a natural product. Laundry detergent, because its

residue, left on clothing, eventually contacts the skin, also should be plain and non-toxic. Facial tissues and toilet paper, since they touch sensitive and absorbent mucous membranes, are also important. Colored and scented varieties treated with chemicals should be avoided. Simple white products are preferable, though much of humanity survives well using cotton handkerchiefs instead of disposable tissues, and water rather than toilet paper. These alternatives are quite hygienic.

Incidentally, since we are for the moment concerned with bathroom matters, we may touch on the issue of body position during the excretory act. The natural position for defecating is the squat, a position which relaxes the intestines and the abdominal muscles. In North America and much (though not all) of Europe, the commode or "sitting toilet" is used. This puts one in a seated position, which however dignified, even regal, is totally unnatural and may even inhibit the excretory act. Fortunately, motivated and/or nimble persons can use standard toilet seats to assume the squatting position. Enough said!

Bathing: Since ancient times human beings have bathed, not just to clean the outside of the body, but to affect it more deeply by relaxing muscles and other soft tissue, and by even changing its biochemical balance. Hot baths, cold baths, and mineral-spring and seawater baths have all been used to promote the health of the body.

The hot bath includes the hot-water bath (as practiced for example in Japan), the Turkish steam bath, and the Scandinavian sauna. These have various benefits. They open the pores and induce perspiration and thus help discharge tissue wastes, excess salts, and liquids. They also help to dissolve excess fats and proteins and, according to some studies, may even help rid the body of heavy metals and chemical pollutants. Hot baths relax the muscles, the nervous system, and the mind. In Japan, nearly every man, woman, and child every day takes a long soak in a hot bath, either at home or in a public facility. The relaxing and regenerative effects of the Japanese *o-furo* ("honorable bath") are extraordinary and I am convinced that much of the ability of the Japanese to survive and thrive under the pressures of modern life is due to its daily use.

The cold-water bath is also a widespread but perhaps less enthusiastically practiced therapeutic device. In Scandinavia the accepted epilogue to a sauna is a roll in the snow or a dip in a frigid lake. In many public baths in Japan there is a small cold tub in a corner of the bathing room. The traditional practice, observed by few people today, is to go back and forth between the cold and the hot tubs. This alternation of Yin and Yang stimulation is supposed to increase circulation, strengthen resistance to cold, and to build "character." One can get a similar but less memorable effect by alternating hot and cold showers.

Seawater bathing has been practiced in many cultures as a form of health maintenance and even therapy. The term *thassalotherapy* refers to seawater therapy. The salinity of seawater is roughly that of human blood and of the intercellular fluid. Also, it contains the trace minerals which the body needs, albeit in minute quantities. Bathing in the sea, then, is like immersion in a giant mineral-supplement solution. The salinity and mineral content of the body is adjusted, with the body giving off excess and taking in what it needs. Bathing in mineral springs is likewise based on the body's ability to absorb beneficial minerals through the skin.

Cold-water ocean bathing is a slightly masochistic but unforgettable form of thassalotherapy. At Boston's "L" Street beach, Brooklyn's Brighton Beach, and at other sacred venues around the world, people immerse themselves daily throughout the year, including during the winter months. Only a person who has actually plunged into thirty-five-degree water while the winter winds whipped sand and snow on the beach can understand the short- and long-term benefits of the experience. The immediate effect is an experience as close to God-consciousness as most of us are likely to enjoy in this lifetime. The permanent effect is a physical and mental hardiness, occasionally tempered by a gnawing and shameful desire to move forever to Miami Beach.

Therapeutic bathing is not for everyone. Ill or debilitated persons must be careful. A short hot bath may relax and revive the less-than-healthy body but a long one will deplete it of important minerals. Cold-water bathing may be too much of a shock to the system. But for most people, properly used baths can help keep the body strong, relaxed, and healthy.

Pace of Life: Thus, for its well-being, the human body requires good nourishment (food, water, air, Ch'i), well-balanced exercise, and also regular cleansing and bathing. But the body, like any living organism, and even most machines, needs to operate at a pace appropriate to itself, and to have periods of rest and recuperation. Thus, a humane pace of life, and regular and refreshing rest and sleep are essential to our health.

There is a certain speed at which the human body functions naturally and comfortably. For example, most people (with the exception of the French) speak at between ninety and one-hundred-twenty words a minute. And most people walk at between two- and three-miles per hour. This natural pace is determined largely by our internal rhythms, by the twelve to fifteen breaths we take per minute, and by the fifty to seventy times our heart beats in that same period. It is determined also by the movements in the natural world around us, by the pace at which a cloud moves across the sky, by the speed at which a river makes its way to the sea. Moving and functioning at this human and humane pace is an important factor in good health. It allows us to be active through the day without becoming physically drained or emotionally exhausted. It allows us to notice and appreciate the myriad small beauties of nature, from a crimson sunset to a wildflower in Spring, and to enjoy the small and subtle pleasures of human life, from a child's greeting to an Elizabethan sonnet.

In pre-industrial times life moved perforce at a relatively slow pace. And today in much of the Third World and in a few, usually rural, parts of the industrialized nations, it still does. This human pace of life persists in a village in India or South America, in an agricultural community in the American south, even in a small town in Britain. But in the cities and suburbs of most of the world, life no longer "creeps in this petty pace." It zooms along at breakneck speed. We move from place to place at speeds inconceivable even a century ago. And once in a place, we perform our tasks at a brisk pace in order to rush on to the next place and task. Many people exist in a state of perpetual rush.

The reason is that our pace of life today is no longer created by human and natural rhythms. It is determined rather by the rate at which machines, mechanical and electronic, operate. We move from place to place in automobiles, buses, trains, and planes. Once arrived, we think, speak, and move to keep pace with the myriad devices designed to save time and effort: electronic cash registers, computers, automatic dishwashers, and microwave ovens. These rapid means of transportation and these labor-saving devices are meant to give us more leisure, more time to relax and enjoy ourselves. Instead they keep us hurtling around, trying to keep pace with them. And when we do "relax" we are likely to do so at the frenetic pace of television sitcom.

The effect on our health and well-being is a negative one. Being moved around as fast as we are, as biological freight in our automobiles, trains, and planes, cannot be very good for us. In an automobile, for example, we are being transported at fifty miles an hour in a metal box, the whole body of which is electrically charged. A few feet away from us in the engine, hundreds of controlled but violent explosions are occurring every second, and temperatures of two to three thousand degrees Fahrenheit are being generated. The effects of automobile travel on the human body have never (as far as I know) been thoroughly studied. I suspect they are substantial. According to the teachings of Anthroposophy, forty miles an hour is the speed at which the *astral* or energetic body begins to separate from the physical body. This is a sobering thought since so many of us spend so much time in automobiles. Travel by jet airplane, which is ten times faster, must be even more disorienting and potentially harmful.

The hurried pace at which we daily function also may be directly harmful to our health. Stress is any factor which prevents an organism from functioning in its natural, normal manner. There are, as we have already discussed, many sources of stress in our lives today: polluted water and air, artificial light, and ionizing radiation. The pace of modern life is another. Much more rapid than our natural and comfortable pace, it keeps our body in a more or less constant state of arousal, in a mild form of the "fight-or-flight" condition. This automatic response allows us in moments of danger to react quickly and forcefully. It involves a rise in blood pressure and in pulse and respiration rates. But the fight-or-flight reaction is meant to be an occasional not a chronic condition, and to be followed by real physical exertion. If it is frequently stimulated, and in situations where extreme physical response is unwarranted, it can impair the natural functioning of the body. Indigestion, muscle tension, and inability to relax and sleep properly may result.

The pace and pressure of life today thus can directly affect us. It can also lead to the use and abuse of prescription and recreational drugs, of everything from alcohol to Darvon to cocaine. There are many factors behind drug use, but an inability to deal with the pressures of modern life is certainly one of them.

It is important then that we slow life to a human and natural pace. Otherwise we may wind up leading full but unnecessarily short lives. One possible measure, popular twenty years ago in the heyday of the "back-to-the-land" movement, is to retreat from the cities and suburbia into the small towns and countryside. But there are other, less radical measures we can take. We do not necessarily have to join the Amish (who abjure modern life and its conveniences totally), or even move to a small town in the middle of Indiana. There are many things we can do to slow down our lives just where we are. For example:

- Choose slower methods of travel. We can go by train or boat rather than plane. On shorter journeys we can go by foot or bicycle rather than automobile. Travel is a process, in which the experience of the movement from one place to another can be as meaningful as the experience of the destination. I suspect that in twenty years there will be a satiation with supersonic travel and a demand for slower alternatives. Quality trains and even oceanic liners will be in demand. Already, bicycle travel has become popular.

- Choose to do things in a slower, but perhaps more relaxing and satisfying manual way rather than an efficient, mechanical one. Mow the lawn with a push mower (yes, they still exist) rather than with a power mower. Cut vegetables with a nicely sharpened knife rather than using a Cuisinart processor. Write a thank you note to someone rather than calling on the phone. Such acts go against our culture's faith, daily reinforced in the advertising media, that faster and easier is necessarily better. But doing something more slowly and with a little effort may give us much more satisfaction. At the least we will get a bit of intrinsic exercise for our trouble.

- Do a daily, one-hour "machine fast." Consciously disconnect from all mechanical and electronic devices, including automobile, telephone, television, and radio, for sixty minutes each day. Read a book, talk to your goldfish, play a game of solitaire. Breathe deeply, talk deliberately, move with deliberation.

- For one day a week observe this same fast. For twenty-four hours, from sunset to sunset perhaps, separate yourself from all the things which are saying, "Faster, faster, hurry up, hurry up!" Put the car in the garage, disconnect the television, give the dishwasher a rest. In the Judeo-Christian world this, of course, is called the Sabbath. It has helped sustain us physically and spiritually for centuries. Unfortunately the legal Sabbath is rapidly disappearing and more and more stores and businesses are open on Sunday. But still on Sunday or Saturday, or any other day, we can unilaterally declare our own day of rest. If God needed his day of leisure after creating the world, we also need ours.

- Once a year, for a week at least, observe the same fast. Stay at home and do "nothing." This is the real meaning of the word "vacation" taken from the French *vacances* or

"emptiness." The trip to Maine with a car full of kids is
nice, but a true fast from machines and their hurried pace
will probably do us more good in the end.

These suggestions bring us into the issue of rest. The human
body, like all other organisms, needs rest, an opportunity to
regenerate and refresh itself. Separating ourselves periodically
from the hubbub of modern life is a way of incorporating real
relaxation and rest into our lives. This art is necessary for our
physical health and for all dimensions of our well-being.

The most total form of rest is sleep, that nightly journey into
the world of dreams which we take after a day of activity. Good
sleep is also essential to health. A moderate diet free of stimu-
lants and chemicals is a necessary first step to good sleep. But
there are a number of other measures that will help insure
proper, restful sleep.

- Have your last meal or snack at least three hours before
  retiring. Going to sleep on a full stomach disturbs both
  digestion and rest.
- Use bed clothes, sheets, and blankets made of natural fibre
  such as 100 percent cotton. And use a mattress stuffed and
  lined with natural materials. The Japanese *futon*, filled with
  cotton batting, is popular today and for good reason. Also,
  use a bed with a wooden frame. During sleep we are re-
  charging with Ch'i and synthetic bedding, mattresses with
  metal springs, and beds with plastic or metal frames, all
  interfere with Ch'i flow.
- If you read or watch television before you sleep, avoid things
  that are too exciting, bizarre, or depressing. Meditative or
  religious writings or poetry are preferable to a war novel,
  a horror movie, or the eleven o'clock news report. Our
  state of mind when we fall asleep can affect our dreams and
  the quality of our sleep.
- Shut off all lights and electrical appliances in the bedroom.
  Do not have an electric clock near your head, and arrange
  the room so that your head is not near an electrical outlet.

Do not sleep with the radio or television on. A non-electric bedroom will permit the free absorption of Ch'i without electromagnetic interference.

• Divide the night's sleep equally around "actual midnight." This is the time midway between sundown and sunset. Thus, if the sun goes down at 6 P.M. and rises at 8 A.M., the actual "middle of the night" is 2 A.M. At this time the Yin quality of the night's Ch'i is strongest. Sleep taken near this time is more deep and restful than sleep taken far from it. Ideally then, a person who sleeps six hours on such a night, will go to bed at eleven and get up at five. Because of the pace of modern life and the ubiquity of electrical lights, we tend to go to bed very late—often close to functional midnight—and to sleep much past it. But the quality of sleep is not so good. The human being is a diurnal creature who should be active in the day and asleep in the middle of the night. It is not easy to maintain this pattern. In the summer, for example, it might involve going to bed at 9 P.M. and rising at 4:30 A.M. But we should keep it in mind as a standard.

Thus a human pace of life, proper rest, and good sleep are very important. Along with proper nourishment from food, water, air, and Ch'i, and with proper hygiene and bathing, they are the basis of physical health. But the health of our physical body is related to each of our other bodies: aesthetic, emotional, intellectual, social, ideological, and spiritual. So these factors are crucial in our overall health and well-being.

Now we must turn to the other dimensions of human life. Each is crucial to the well-being of the entire organism. We must explore how, from the Macrobiotic point of view, each can be nourished and exercised to promote its own health and that of the organism as a whole.

3. Feasting with the Senses

Taste is the *only* morality. Tell me what you like
and I will tell you what you are.
Life without industry is guilt; industry without art
is brutality.

John Ruskin (1819–1900)

Some years ago a friend and I were traveling in a remote part of
Japan. After a long train ride we arrived one evening in a small
town and were directed to the local inn or *ryokan*. A wooden
building in the traditional style, with a red tile roof and a wooden
wall around it, it seemed from the outside a modest but pleasant
place. Within however, past the sliding doors of polished wood
at the main entrance, it was a world of simple, magical beauty.
The floors and pillars were all of the same gleaming, dark wood.
The walls were of white plaster, inset here and there with screens
of latticed bamboo. In an interior courtyard was a small, im-
maculate garden, with artfully arranged dwarf pines and white
stones, through which passed a small stream. An elderly woman,
with steel-gray hair combed neatly back and wearing a *kimono*
of indigo blue, greeted us with a bow and softly spoken words
of welcome and respect. As she led us to our room there was no
sound, but the murmur of flowing water and the shuffle of our
now-slippered feet.

Our room was spacious, with yielding gold-yellow *tatami*, or
reed mats, covering the floor. One set of sliding doors was open
to reveal the view of the garden. In an alcove at the far end was
a hanging scroll depicting a hawk in full-winged flight. Beneath
the painting was an arrangement of flowers in a squat blue vase.
Everything was spotlessly clean. Freshly laundered and starched
yukata (evening kimono) of blue and white had been laid out for
us. After a hot soak in the *o-furo* we donned the yukata and sat
down to dinner in the room. The meal was brought in by several
young women, each attired in a colorful silk kimono, and moving
with quiet and consummate grace and discretion. Each course,

presented on a small but lovely dish, was a study in form and
color as well as taste.

After a time, warmed and expansive from the thimblefuls of
warm *saké* (rice wine) we had drunk, my friend and I leaned
back and beheld in silence the scene around us. From across the
tiled rooftops of the neighboring houses came the delicate strains
of a *shamisen* or Japanese harp, interwoven with the fragrance
of incense from a Buddhist altar somewhere nearby. Thus augmented, the beauty and harmony of the room enclosed and
transported us. The outside world and our missions, duties, and
troubles in it vanished. Past and future vanished. The setting
and the moment became the vessel for a dimensionless peace.
We slept that night the sleep of angels. The next morning we
left, refreshed and smiling, albeit with a touch of regret.

Two days later we arrived very late in a small, but busy coastal
city. After some difficulty we found a room in a "business hotel"
which caters to traveling salesmen. It was a four-story concrete
box with linoleum floors of bright red and green, and with rooms,
hallways, and even bath illuminated with glaring fluorescent lights.
Our room was like a cheap 1950's American motel room which
had been shrunk to one-third size. It smelled of tobacco smoke
and mold. In the dining room, an indifferent and sweaty man in
a soiled apron plunked down before us an indifferent (but we
hoped not sweaty) meal. Loud, raucous music blared from
a television directly over our heads. Frazzled and exhausted
from the day, we went to bed, only to discover that our room
faced on a highway. Although we slept, our sleep and dreams
were punctuated all night by the throaty roar of heavy trucks.
In the morning, we made an early getaway, frazzled and still
tired, anxious only to get to a more congenial spot by lunch time.

These two experiences, in the old inn and in the business
hotel, represent extremes perhaps, but they illustrate a principle:
our sensory experiences vary tremendously and can have a significant effect on us. The things we see, hear, touch, smell, and
taste, influence directly our sense organs, but affect as well every
aspect of our being.

Our five senses keep us informed about what is going on in

our immediate environment. Our sense of taste judges substances from the external world (usually food and drink) that we actually take into our mouths. There, taste buds embedded in the tongue judge their particular quality. Our sense of touch, located in the nerve endings of the skin, judges things with which we come into contact. We feel the air, or touch a stone or piece of cloth, and we can tell whether it is hot or cold, smooth or rough, moving or still. Our sense of smell is located high in the nasal passages. It is a small mucous-covered area in which are imbedded bundles of nerve fibres. It is sensitive to the air-born molecules of aromatic substances—woodsmoke, benzene, wildflowers. Even a few such aromatic molecules coming in contact with this area stimulate the olfactory nerve. Our sense of hearing responds to vibrations from an oscillating body such as the human vocal cords, a drum head, or an electrical motor. These vibrations are picked up by the external ear. They are then directed through the ear canal to the tiny, sensitive bones of the inner ear. The vibration is passed to the nerves and thence to the brain. And our sense of sight is sensitive to light (the visible range of the electromagnetic spectrum) originating from or reflected off objects around us. With it we can distinguish the form and color of things six inches or six miles away.

Thus, through our five senses, we gather information about the external world. We are doing this all the time. Even when we sleep our senses are at work. Hence we start into wakefulness if there is a loud noise, a bright light, or even a very strong odor. And throughout our waking hours, even though we are not always aware of it, our senses are bringing in impressions. A man reading the newspaper on his back porch feels the summer breeze on his cheek, smells the roses in the garden, and hears the songs of birds, even though his attention is quite elsewhere. And likewise, a person walking on a street in Manhattan is receiving the noise, smell, and images of the environment even though he is daydreaming and paying no attention to them.

This sensory data, consisting of sights, sounds, aromas, tastes, and tactile sensations, are a kind of "food." Like the food we eat, it is ingested, it becomes part of us, and it has a profound effect on the condition of the whole organism. Sometimes we are acutely aware of the effect of this sensory "food." A magnificent mountain view sends us into a peaceful, meditative reverie. An evening in a Japanese inn, such as that enjoyed by my friend and I, transports us out of the mundane world to the borders of the transcendent. Or the sights and sounds of a highway strip make us depressed and sick to our stomach. Usually though, we are not aware of the effects of the sensory impressions, as we are often unaware of the impressions themselves. But they are coming into us all the time, nevertheless. And they are influencing us in every dimension of our being. This food which we take in through our senses of touch, smell, hearing, sight is a major factor in our health and well-being.

Part of this sensory food is "natural," having been created by Mother Nature. She is an unfailing multimedia artist. Each element of her works of art, each line and color, texture, sound, and fragrance is beautiful in itself. And she combines them in a harmonious and synergistic way to create a stunning comprehensive beauty. In a high mountain environment, for example, the vista of land and sky, the sound of wind and running water, the fragrance of soil, flower, and grass, the warmth of the sun, and the soft yielding of the earth underfoot together comprise a flawless, magnificent *objet d'art*. Sometimes, to be sure, even Mother Nature stretches the canons of good taste (at least from a human standard). It is hard for us to appreciate, for example, the face of a bat or the aroma of a skunk. But in almost all her works, large and small, there is an unmistakable beauty. It is a beauty which rests the body, calms the mind, and elevates the spirit. And it is a beauty to which instinctively, we turn for comfort in moments of trouble.

A human-made environment may be a beautiful, aesthetically pleasing one. We human beings can design and build beautiful homes, surround them with lovely gardens, furnish them with fine carpets, furniture, and decorations, fill them with music and even with refreshing scents. We have an instinct and an ability to instill beauty into all our creations. And we are able even on a large scale to create venues which can compare with the creations of nature—witness Paris, Dresden, and Kyoto of little more than a century ago.

Unfortunately, we lack Mother Nature's consistency and her limitless resources. Sometimes our aesthetic sense goes awry, and sometimes, quite often in fact, it is sacrificed to economy and function. So we create things which either are aesthetically neutral or are in fact repulsive to our sight, hearing, smell, and touch. Into the world comes a row of tract houses, the rattle of a chain saw, and the sterile feel of cold vinyl. Such sensory "food" dismays rather than pleases, enervates rather than nourishes us. It can undermine the health of body, mind, and spirit.

In the pre-industrial world, when good taste failed, or economic necessity triumphed, the resulting aesthetic affront was usually limited in scope. Medieval London, for example, was in some ways a difficult place to live. It was crowded, muddy, and to be blunt, it smelled bad. Yet its street life was vital and colorful, and its architecture had a rugged simple beauty still evident today in The Tower of London. Also, with its narrow streets, low buildings and a total area of less than two square miles, it was a city built on a human scale. And it was surrounded by field, forest and river. In the late 20th century we have the ability to devastate the natural world and to erect vast artificial environments. A housing project of today is likely miles from any unspoiled environment, and its sullen concrete towers can hardly be called picturesque.

What we create is sometimes impressive, from a distance at least, such as New York City with its magnificent skyline. But more often it is not. Our urban and suburban environments stretch for miles, dominated by boxlike buildings of concrete and steel, by asphalt streets and highways, by power lines and billboards, by the roar of traffic and by the smell of engine exhaust. The natural world, remains in remnant only, in an occasional tree, patch of grass, or park. The interiors of this environment are also apt to be quite sterile. Very likely they are dominated by straight lines, right angles, plastic materials, monochrome, slick surfaces, and glaring lights.

The result is that many of us today are deprived of contact with the nourishing beauty of nature, and are immersed in an unattractive, at best aesthetically neutral, artificial environment. We are so used to the situation that we take it for granted. We are not aware of its immediate and long-term effects. But it is affecting us moment to moment, day to day, in obvious and in subtle ways. For example, loud mechanical noises, such as that of a jet plane passing overhead, shock the nervous system and stimulate the fight-or-flight response. Though we are scarcely aware of it, our body tenses, and our pulse and respiration rate and our blood pressure rise. Studies of people living in the flight path of Los Angeles International Airport indicate a much higher than normal incidence of nervous and emotional disorders. Someday perhaps, studies will indicate what effect a rectilinear, plastic and steel environment has on the human organism.

It is important then, that we have good sensory "food" everyday. Of course we exercise little or no control over the general environment. If we live in an unattractive and noisy part of a city, we can, if we have the means, move to the country or to a well-to-do suburb. Or we can wear dark glasses and carry a Walkman to protect ourselves from the bombardment of the senses. But generally speaking, we are stuck with it. We do however have control over our home and perhaps over our workplace. There we can create an environment which nourishes and stimulates the senses in a positive way.

We are faced then with the question: "What kind of environment should we try to create?" With what forms and colors, textures, sounds, and even aromas should we surround ourselves? Aesthetic preferences vary according to our background and individuality. But four principles are generally valid: naturalness, simplicity, order, and cleanliness.

Naturalness: We are creatures of nature and we instinctively yearn for the images and colors, the textures, and other sense stimuli of the natural world. We cannot, we need not, replicate nature in our interior environments. But we should keep in mind the aesthetics of the world around us. The lines and forms of nature are fluid and graceful, her colors are usually muted and mixed—with greens, browns, grays, blues, and reds blended harmoniously in every surface. There are few monochromatic phenomenon. Even a perfectly blue sky usually has varying shades of color. The sounds of nature are soft and unobtrusive and her aromas subtle and inoffensive.

Of course, if we use natural materials such as stone, wood, and cotton in the construction, furnishing, and decoration of our homes, this natural aesthetic will be easily achieved. And if we use materials which are from the local environment, we can realize even an "ecologically appropriate" aesthetic. The traditional architecture and interior design of every pre-modern, pre-industrial culture reflect this impulse.

It is possible today to adopt and even develop these traditional "natural" patterns. Anthroposophical interior design, for example, attempts to do this. It relies on natural materials. It prefers subtly curving, organic lines to straight edges and right angles. Door frames, windows, tables and chairs, are all characterized by graceful curving lines. The walls are painted not with a single color but with several shades of one color or with several different colors which blend into one another. Since colors are understood to have a particular and powerful effect on our body, emotions, and mind, the color of each room is carefully selected. Wall hangings and paintings reflect this same sensitivity and inclination to the natural. The net result is an indoor environment that nourishes all the senses and the human being as a whole.

Natural objects, especially living ones, help create a "natural" interior environment. In Japan, most people live in crowded cities where the nearest remnant of nature may be miles away. Yet they manage to retain the reality and spirit of nature. Most homes and even apartments, however tiny they may be, have a garden. It may be only a few square feet, but it will contain a tiny tree or two, bushes and flowers, some stones, perhaps even a small pool of running water. If there is no garden there will likely be a *bonsai*, or potted dwarfed tree with a few stones and a bit of moss at its base. The Japanese use their gardens and bonsai as objects of contemplation and as sources of inspiration and consolation. Since all the elements of nature are present, though on a small scale, the harmony and power of the macrocosm are present as well. We should remember that in any living or working space, however modest, it is possible with potted plants, a well-chosen stone, or a piece of polished wood, to retain contact with the natural world.

Few of us have the resources to design and build our home from the ground up. And few of us even have the resources to transform our interior environment completely. But we can gradually introduce furnishings and decorations, handmade perhaps, of wood, ceramic, cotton, wool, and other natural materials. We can replace what is plastic, mass-produced, monochromatic, and gaudy. This process may involve expense and inconvenience, but it is well worth it. Our surroundings are food for us, an important source of nourishment. They are affecting us physically, emotionally, mentally every day. And here, as in the choice of food to eat, buying cheap is generally a false economy. It is better to have a few things of quality, than many which are second-rate.

Simplicity: In nature every element is both functional and beautiful. Each stone, plant, tree, and mountain contributes to the life of the whole and to its aesthetic harmony. There is a "simplicity" then in the natural world, which our interior environments should have as well. They should include only those things which are useful and/or aesthetically pleasing.

Unfortunately, we human beings have a very strong "chipmunk" instinct. That is, we acquire things, use them and appreciate them. But when they are no longer useful or attractive we hold on to them. We become, to put it bluntly, junk collectors. Old magazines, books in which we have no interest, tattered, out-of-style clothing, worn-out tools, machines which do not work, and dead batteries fill our living space and spill over into dim and hidden storage areas. Unwilling to let go of something from the past, afraid to be caught unequipped perhaps in an unforeseen emergency, we hold on to the material effluvia of our lives.

To create a healthy living environment we must overcome this "chipmunk instinct." Each object we have around us has a vibratory field or "energy." If the object is used and appreciated this energy is positive and adds to the vitality of the environment and of the people in it. If the object is neither used nor appreciated, its energy becomes negative. This negative "field" reduces the vital force in an environment. Even things hidden in closets and attics are affecting the energy of a home or work-place. To simplify an environment, to clear it of clutter and junk, is to make it much more a positive and healthful place to be.

Simplicity is important in itself. But it is important also in that it makes the qualities of order and cleanliness easier to achieve.

Order: The objects in a given space can be arranged to create a sense of order and balance. In designing an interior environment we create this order intuitively, establishing a balance between space empty and space filled, between horizontal and vertical lines. A well-arranged room when it is "in order" conveys a feeling of peace and well-being. Of course, the main problem then is to maintain the order. Things are used, and left where they have been used. Slowly, ineluctably, in accordance with the Second Law of Thermodynamics, any inhabited space moves away from order toward chaos. The pattern of the sensory stimuli it gives to the people in it changes, and "disorder" rather than "order" is transmitted. It is important then to maintain order, to keep things in their places. In a simple, uncluttered environment, this is easier to do than in one brimming with "collectables."

Cleanliness: Dirt and dust accumulate, literally out of "thin air." They can cover and in effect "hide" within a few days the natural, simple, and orderly environment we have taken such trouble to create. Thus it is important to dust (preferably with a moist cloth), sweep, and mop our living and working environment, regularly, preferably daily. Again, if our home is a simple one, this will be a much easier, quicker task.

In Japan, one of the universal customs is that of *o-soji* or "honorable cleaning." In homes, shops, schools, and factories, and especially in monasteries and other places for spiritual development, *o-soji* usually starts the day. Everything is swept, dusted, and mopped until it gleams and radiates. Unimpeded by dust and dirt, the Ch'i in the house and environs is free to circulate. The Japanese believe that not only is the environment made clean and pure, but that the body, mind, and heart of those cleaning are also purified. A Zen proverb observes, "To polish the floor is to polish one's innermost Mind."

A natural, tasteful, simple, orderly, and clean environment is thus an important factor in our health and well-being. It helps us to be energetic, active, and clear-headed every day, to resist disease, and even to cure ourselves when ill. (Cleanliness is a high priority in the room of a sick person.) The creation and conscientious maintenance of such an environment is as important in the Macrobiotic way of life as eating a proper diet.

My famous (well not too famous, only seven people know about it at the present time) "One Day Cure for Anemia, Swollen Ankles, Weltschmerz—and Anything Else That Ails You," is a practical application of this interrelationship between ourselves and our surroundings. It is based on the fact that we create our environment, which in turn deeply influences us, and that therefore, if we are sick, we can help cure ourselves by changing the environment. The famous "One-Day Cure" includes the following famous steps:

1. Take stock of how you feel, physically and mentally: "crummy," "bad," "horrendous," or "death's door."
2. Take stock of your personal environment—room, apartment, or house. Classify it as "a little ragged," "messy," "catastrophic," or "chimpanzee plus."
3. Remind yourself that condition and environment are creating each other and that you can break the cycle.

4. Start to clean and simplify. Sometimes things are in such
a state of disorder that one hardly knows where to begin.
The kitchen is a good place to start. Wash and dry the
inevitable pile of dirty dishes. Empty the refrigerator.
Throw out the mold-encrusted remnants of last week's
dinner and the jar of mustard whose contents have turned
blue. Clean the pantry and consolidate its contents. Move
on to the living room. Collect and discard old newspapers
and magazines; gather the dirty clothing, and put it into
a laundry bag. When all the rooms have been thus super-
ficially purged, then dust, sweep, vacuum, and mop. Be
thorough. Get those dust balls from under the couch. Then
take all the dirty laundry to the laundromat. If there is
nothing clean to wear, put on a raincoat. While the
laundry is washing, drive to a car wash, avoiding the
police vice squad on route. They are usually on the look-
out for people in raincoats and bare legs. Give your car
a thorough cleaning inside and out. Once home with your
clean laundry, carefully put it away. Take a hot bath and
put on some fresh clean clothing.

5. Sit down for a moment. Survey your beautiful home and
notice how good you already feel. Congratulate yourself,
but do not become complacent. You are not quite through.
"The Great Purge" yet remains.

6. Carry out "The Great Purge," also known in some circles
as "The Materialist's Enema." Go to your clothing closet.
Survey what hangs therein and ask yourself: Is there
anything here which I have not worn in the past six months
and probably will not wear in the next six? Very likely
the answer will be yes. You may have (as I do) an orange
colored T-shirt which says "I love Dubuque" across the
chest. Given to you by your great aunt Hilda, this shirt
has never been worn. You keep it, though, thinking that
perhaps some day you will be invited to a party in Iowa
and the dress requirement will be just such an orange
treasure. Take the shirt and other extraneous items and
put them in a large cardboard box. (A plastic bag will do

as well but is less ecological.) Repeat this selection process in your kitchen, at your bookcase, and at other strategic points where junk accumulates. You may discover a rusted omelet pan unused for a decade, a book on composting techniques in nineteenth century Lithuania, a cracked tennis racquet with no strings. Deposit these objects and all other clutter in the "TO GO" box. Take this box to an appropriate destination—to a secondhand charity store, to the town dump, or if you are in a vengeful mood, to the home of your dearest enemy—and unburden yourself of it.

Parting with effluvia can be a difficult, painful, even traumatic experience. When it is over, however, you will be amazed and gratified. Your home will seem remarkably cleaner, brighter, and more peaceful. And you will feel as if you had just laid down a sixty-pound backpack.

7. (Optional) On the way home buy yourself something as a reward, preferably something consumable, such as a bottle of fine wine, or living, such as a new plant.

8. Sit down again. Survey with pride the effect of your work. Sip your wine. Talk to your new plant. Listen to a piece of fine music. Relax. Then schedule your next purge. Human nature being what it is, this will be necessary between three days and six months in the future.

9. If by this time you are not feeling great, start from step one again. Focus on closets, the attic, the garage, cellar, and other loci of cosmic junk accumulations. This second effort can often lead to many hours or even days of purging. The effect is proportionally profound. There is a tribe in Africa, a smart one and probably a healthy and happy one, which has a notable attitude to material possessions. Each year the members put all their moveable property (it is to be sure not very much) on a raft, ignite the raft and set it adrift. Such extreme custom may be impractical in our society but it can teach us something.

Naturalness, order, simplicity, and cleanliness are relevant
also to that movable house which protects us from the environment, the clothes we choose to wear every day. Our clothes influence profoundly how we feel and think. Regardless of their
style and level of formality, they should be orderly and simple.
And they should be freshly laundered. Clothing picks up dust,
dirt and pollutants which reduce its Ch'i. It needs to be cleaned
and refreshed to regain its native energy. Clothes which have
been worn for a day or more become "tired," and need washing
even if they are not patently dirty. If we wear "tired" clothes
we will be affected by their "tiredness." Laundering is not just
cleaning, it is a baptism, a purification which is passed on to us
through our clothing. Our clothing, like our living environment,
reflects our condition but also creates it. Clothes do indeed
"make the man."

Art: The term "art" comes from the Greek word *artunein* which
means to "arrange." In the "fine arts," (painting, drawing,
sculpture, architecture, and ceramics), and in the musical arts
(music, song, and dance), sensory stimuli are "arranged" in order
to produce a strong and specific effect. The creations of some
arts, of architecture and ceramics, for example, can have a practical as well as aesthetic aim. The creations of the others, though,
are purely aesthetic. Their *raison d'etre* is the stimulation and
pleasing of the senses. All works of art, however, while profoundly affecting the senses, affect all other dimensions of the
human being as well. Thus buildings, pieces of ceramic, paintings,
drawings, sculpture, and works of music, can play a major role
in our lives.

In his book, *The Secret Power of Music* (Inner Traditions,
Rochester, Vermont, 1986), Englishman David Tame presents
the following opinion. Music is the vibration of the air, ordered
and arranged in a particularly powerful manner. It is a form of
energy then, one which has been shown to profoundly affect
plants and animals as well as human beings. Its effect on human
beings is very great. Music can directly affect the different

chakras or "energy centers" of the human organism and thus influence physical processes, emotions, thoughts, patterns of behavior, morality, and even spiritual consciousness.

There is a particularly close connection between music and morality, Tame observes, which has long been recognized. Plato emphasized the importance of proper music in forming the ethical human being. And in ancient China the emperors carefully monitored the music played in their domains. They believed that on it hinged the morality and morale of the populace. Some types of music, including Western classical music (particularly of the seventeenth and eighteenth centuries), manifest in their rhythms and harmonics certain universal patterns. This music has an ordering, harmonizing, and moralizing effect on those who listen to it. According to Tame, other types of music including rock-and-roll, most jazz, and much of contemporary serious music (atonal music, electronic music) pervert the archetypal patterns. Such music confuses the mind and moral sense, and inclines the listener to bestiality and immorality. Tame attributes the moral and social decline of the West largely to the evil influence of modern, popular music.

Tame overstates his case perhaps. The consciousness and morality of a culture certainly are influenced by the music it experiences. But that music is to some degree an expression of the changing consciousness of the culture. The two create and influence each other. And there are other factors affecting both consciousness and music, including developments in diet, technology, philosophy, and in the other arts.

His basic point though, is well taken. Music is an important factor in our individual and collective lives. It is a kind of "food"—a consciously prepared or "cooked" set of auditory stimuli. Music obviously affects our aesthetic body, but it affects as well all the other dimensions of our being. Music can change our physical processes, emotions, desires, and thoughts.

The same is true of the creations of the other arts—of paintings, sculpture, drawings, and pottery. These are a visual "food," which use form, line, and color to affect the sense of sight. Similarly, their actual affect is upon the entire organism. As I am a changed person after listening to Beethoven's Eroica symphony, I am also a changed person after contemplating Rembrandt's "Descent from the Cross," or Rodin's "The Thinker."

Different works of art affect us in different ways. All directly affect the aesthetic body, but each in addition strongly influences one or more of the other bodies. For example, certain types of rock-and-roll especially stimulate the physical body. Love songs and romantic music affect the emotional body. And church music, a Bach cantata, for example, especially affects the moral and spiritual dimension. The influence of a work of art can be either strong or weak. It can also be harmonizing, nourishing, and refining, or it can be disruptive and disorienting. Thus, I am a different person after listening to Verdi's *Requiem* than I am after listening to an album of "heavy metal" popular music. And I am a different person after driving down a "fast food strip" than I am after contemplating the beauty of Notre Dame cathedral. The effects of art upon us are real, specific, and substantial.

We should then exercise care in selecting the art to which we expose ourselves. We must choose the music we listen to and the paintings and drawings we look at with the same discernment we use in choosing our daily food. We need to seek out those aesthetic experiences which will influence us in the way we wish to be influenced. This is important to our general health and well-being.

Fortunately, there is a vast resource of art from which to chose this aesthetic "food." Each culture has produced many works of art. Some were produced by its sophisticated elite, some by its common folk. And each culture has treasured those works which most directly and powerfully nourish, in a positive way, the aesthetic and other human bodies. Thus nearly every major culture has preserved a classical and a folk heritage, consisting of that music, painting, sculpture, dance, and pottery which most pleased the senses, stirred the emotions, refined the moral consciousness, and elevated the mind and spirit of its people.

Today we are privileged to have access to a vast range of this artistic heritage. The treasures of far-off times and places, of Greece in the sixth century B.C., and of Africa in the thirteenth century, as well as of our own culture and era, are known to us. And they are easily accessible. Phonograph records, compact discs, museum prints, and art books bring to us cheaply and at our convenience great works of art (or at least their facsimile) from all lands and ages. Art galleries, museums, exhibitions, and concerts present these works in their original form. Thus we can enjoy the sitar ragas of Indian music, the landscapes of Van Gogh, the architecture of early New England, the dance of Thailand, almost when and where we wish. We can easily tap the vast legacy of human creativity to nourish our aesthetic and other bodies as we would like to nourish them. And we can thereby contribute to our health and happiness.

However, the art which immediately surrounds us is mostly contemporary and commercial, rather than classical or folk. This includes the visual images which assault us from every billboard, magazine advertisement, and television commercial, as well as serious modern art. It includes most music on the radio, in elevators and supermarkets—"hard rock," "soft rock," "rock rock," "schmaltz," and "Muzak,"—as well as the work of serious composers. It includes mass-produced trinkets and ornaments as well as the work of skilled craftspersons. Some of this art is elevating and inspiring. It may, in time, be recognized as truly nourishing "great art." It may become part of our classical or folk artistic heritage. But much is trivial, superficial, and ineffectual, and contributes little to our happiness or health. It disappears and deservedly so after a month or a year.

We have, then, spread before us a rich and varied smorgasbord of art from which to nourish ourselves. It contains the works of the classical and folk traditions of many cultures and times. It includes also the largely ephemeral products of our own time and place. We can and should sample from the latter. We are creatures of the contemporary world and should be in touch with it. But we should perhaps draw most of our nourishment from the music, art, dance, of our proven heritage. We will benefit more from listening to Mozart than to Madonna, and more from placing on our office wall a Turner seascape rather than a velveteen painting of large-eyed bunnies.

This approach to art may seem elitist. And indeed it is. But a diet, which excludes white bread, "TV Dinners," and Mac-Donald hamburgers in favor of whole grains, fresh organic vegetables and fruits, is also elitist. One involves choosing the best food for the physical body, and the other involves choosing the best "food" for the aesthetic body. A selective approach to food and to art may be elitist but it is also prudent and wise.

Our aesthetic food, like our daily edible food, must be consumed carefully and consciously. However, we are so surrounded and bombarded by music and other artistic stimuli, that we take them for granted. We seldom give them our undivided attention. So when Mozart across the centuries invites us to listen to his opera "The Magic Flute," a magnificent product of his human insight, musical genius, and hard labor, we reply "Why thank you, Wolfgang, how very kind! But would you mind if I wash my car at the same time?" Poor Wolfgang. Poor Opera. Poor us. We derive only a fraction of the benefit from that masterpiece that we might. And similarly, we go to the museum and pass through a roomful of paintings by Monet while chatting with a friend about our summer plans. We listen to Brahms and read the evening paper. We have a Japanese woodblock print on the wall and forget that it is there. In other words, we come to the table of art but we bolt our food and miss the real pleasure and benefit of eating.

We need to chew our daily (edible) food very well to get the maximum benefit from it. Likewise, we need to chew our carefully selected aesthetic food very well. It is good, then, from time to time to give a work of art our undivided attention. To sit in a quiet and darkened room and to listen to Wagner's "Lohengrin," to contemplate Picasso's "Guernica" for an uninterrupted hour, or to hold, carefully inspect, and with one's fingertips explore a piece of fine pottery can be a profound and transforming experience.

We can immerse ourselves, as well, in the works of that consummate artist, Mother Nature. There are many simple sense-awareness exercises that will open us to the manifold beauty around us. For example, we can for twenty minutes focus on a single stone, or square foot of tree bark. Or we can sit for a period in a wood or on the beach with eyes closed and listen intently to the myriad sounds. We can blindfold ourselves and explore with our hands the shapes and textures of a stone, tree, plant, even a patch of soil. These same exercises can be used with human-made objects, a book, brick wall, or bicycle, not meant to be objects of art, but having nonetheless aesthetic value.

This careful and conscious appreciation of art, whether it be the creation of nature, of craftspersons, or of great artists, nourishes, enriches, and transforms the body, mind, and spirit. It is a necessary part of the Macrobiotic diet and the Macrobiotic way of life.

The appreciation of art is important, but the creation of art is equally important. Nature effortlessly and ceaselessly produces pleasing sights, sounds, textures, and aromas. We, as creatures of nature, also have an ability to create things of beauty. And we must exercise it to become full and healthy human beings.

From the dawn of history and before, human beings have exhibited the desire and the skill to bring beauty into the world. Forty thousand years ago in France, artists decorated the walls of caves with magnificent murals of the hunt. And since then every known human culture has, in making the necessities of life—bowls, baskets, clothing, and houses—gone beyond the purely functional. Each has injected beauty in form, color, and texture into its creations. And each culture has also manifested beauty in nonfunctional creations—in its music, dance, and other arts.

The human aesthetic impulse and capability, instinctive and universal, is present in every normal healthy child. Any five-year-old given a lump of clay will start to form it into a pleasing shape. That same child hearing music will start to move its body in harmony with it. The desire and the ability to create beauty is present also in every adult, though it may be suppressed and undeveloped. Every human being is by nature a craftsperson and an artist.

In the pre-industrial world most people could express this part of their nature. Since all things were made by hand, each artisan (smith, carpenter, seamstress) could in his craft express his aesthetic sense. Besides, music, song, and dance were part of the regular, even daily life of the community, in which every man, woman, and child participated. For example, even today, aboriginal peoples (whom we have the curious audacity to label "primitive") spend about twenty percent of their waking hours singing and dancing. In literate cultures, the genuinely cultured person was expected to be accomplished in the creative and performing arts as well as the literary ones. The Chinese Confucian scholar, for example, knew the literary "Classics," but he could also play the lute, write and recite poetry, and paint. The English gentleperson of the last century was likewise accomplished in the arts. Thus, while the common folk were singing and dancing on the village green, the women and men in the manor house were painting, singing, and staging dramatic productions.

Today the situation is quite different. The opportunity for aesthetic expression in most jobs is minimal. Products are designed by one or several persons and then manufactured by machines. The true craftsperson, creating useful objects of beauty, is rare. And the active participation in art has become the domain of the very few. Most of us have become passive consumers of art, rather than its creators and performers.

Behind this situation is an insidious idea—that the world consists of two types of people: those able to create art and those able only to consume it. The first is a small, gifted elite whose profession is to write novels and poems, paint pictures, direct and act in theatre and cinema, and create sculpture. The second group includes the rest of us, the fumble-fingered, tone-deaf, and color-blind who were in the shower when the good Lord was giving out artistic talent. Our role is to consume what is produced by the gifted professionals. Hence, if we wish to experience music we turn on the radio or we buy a record. If we wish to experience visual art we go to the museum or buy a print. If we wish to experience dance we go to the ballet, or watch a televised performance.

The appreciation of art is important to human life. But it is only one-half of the artistic enterprise. We can enjoy the creations of others, but we must also create things of beauty ourselves. The impulse to create beauty is a deep and powerful one. If cultivated and developed it will give great and daily pleasure and satisfaction. It will contribute to our total health and well-being. If neglected it will be a source of frustration and dissatisfaction that will hurt us physically, emotionally, and psychologically.

Thus we must each (if we are not already) become artists and performers. Our schools do not educate us for this. Music and art are the poor sisters of the academic world. The last exposure many people have is finger painting in the fourth grade. And the media, serving the needs of the consumer economy, encourage us to be consumers rather than creators of art. But nevertheless we can recover and cultivate the artist, the craftperson, the singer, or the dancer who is in each of us.

There are many opportunities in our daily life to express artistic creativity. In decorating a home, in choosing a wardrobe, in preparing and presenting a meal, even in simply speaking or moving, we can either manifest harmony and beauty or fail to. Most of us, by devoting a little more time and effort, could greatly enrich these daily activities. And we would be greatly enriched in return. We are all by necessity multi-media artists as we present ourselves in the world. We might as well make the most of it.

Besides these aesthetic activities intrinsic to life, there are crafts and also pure arts. Crafts produce objects that are useful as well as beautiful and thus include pottery, weaving, sewing, carpentry, and furniture making. Pure arts are *ars qratia ars*, "art for its own sake," and thus include painting, drawing, music, sculpture, and dance.

Every human being can practice some "extrinsic" art or craft with reasonable accomplishment. Even so-called handicapped and retarded people can develop high levels of skill and creativity. We may not achieve a professional level, but that is not important. What is important is that we develop and regularly use whatever ability we do have. Many people go through life wishing they had studied the piano or learned to dance, or to knit. They feel a deep frustration, one which may affect their emotional and even physical health.

The practice and even mastery of a craft or art can begin at any age. "Grandma Moses," the noted painter, began painting when she was past retirement age. It is never too late. And fortunately, the opportunities for training in our society are almost limitless. School and community college evening courses, YMCA-YWCA classes, accomplished friends and neighbors, how-to books and cassettes are all available to the motivated person.

Compared to the other duties and tasks with which life is filled, cultivating an art or craft may not seem important. But along with creating a simple, natural, clean and orderly environment, and with being careful in our choice of artistic stimuli, being artistically creative is necessary for the health of the aesthetic body. And since this body affects our general health, all three pursuits are essential to our happiness and well-being. Hence all three are essential parts of the Macrobiotic way of life.

4. Secrets of the Laughing Buddha

Happiness is the only sanction of life; where happiness fails, existence remains a mad and lamentable experiment.

George Santayana (1863–1952)

Related to our physical and aesthetic bodies, but also distinct from them, is our emotional body. This experiences the various "affects" or emotions. There are many different emotions. Some, such as anger, joy, and despair, are states of high arousal with clear and intense characteristics. Others, such as contentment and restlessness, are quite subtle. Some emotions, such as jealousy and affection, have a specific external object. Others, such as peacefulness and anxiety, have no specific object. Some, such as love and anticipation, are positive, in that they are pleasant and energizing. Others, such as fear and hate, are negative, in that they are unpleasant and can interfere with our functioning.

Our emotions are constantly changing. In a single day, in a single hour, even in a single minute, we experience a variety of emotions, subtle and intense, specific and diffuse, positive and negative. Despite this changeability, our emotional body has an abiding inclination or "personality" created by the types of emotions prevalent in it. According to the intensity of its responses, the emotional body will be either "intense" or "low key." According to whether its emotions are in response to external, specific stimuli, or to internal ones, it will be "introverted" or "extroverted." And according to the positive or negative quality of its reactions, it will be "happy" or "unhappy."

The healthy emotional body is the happy one. It is characterized by a predominance of positive emotions. They may be intense (joy, rapture, ecstasy) or subtle (anticipation, amusement), inner-directed (contentment, self-respect) or outer-directed (affection, love), but they must be positive. Or course, even the healthy emotional body experiences negative emotions—such as fear, anger, and guilt. These are an inevitable part of life. But in the emotionally healthy person they play only a minor role. They serve as a subtle and manageable counterpoint to the dominant positive emotions.

There are various factors affecting our emotional body and what it experiences. It is intimately connected with our more Yang or materialized aspects—the physical and aesthetic bodies—and with our more Yin or spiritualized dimensions—the intellectual, moral, and spiritual. And it is easily affected by those other bodies. For example, six martinis in one evening will probably leave me depressed the next morning, and a rigorous six-mile run may cure that very depression. Discovering a sun-drenched field of daisies on a morning stroll will no doubt brighten my spirits, just as reading a book on the destruction of the tropical rain forests may dampen them.

But this relationship between our emotions and the other dimensions of our life is reciprocal. Our emotional body is affecting our physical body, our thoughts, and our spiritual condition. *The Yellow Emperor's Classic of Internal Medicine*, the source-book of Chinese medicine, observes that a person with weak kidneys will be prone to anxiety and worry. But it also observes that a person whose life is filled with anxiety-producing circumstances is likely to develop weak kidneys. So our emotional body is active and influential, as well as passive and responsive. While affected by the physical, aesthetic, and other bodies, it generates its own emotional energy, which in turn influences all aspects of our being. Thus a person who is deeply in love often has great physical and mental energy. Someone grieved by the death of a loved one is probably listless and confused.

Emotional health depends in part on the intelligent cultivation of the other aspects of life—on eating a good diet, getting adequate exercise, on leading a rich aesthetic life, on developing positive mental attitudes. But it depends also on the proper nourishment and exercise of the emotional body.

There are many factors which are directly crucial to emotional health. They include:

- Self-acceptance
- Fulfillment of vocation
- Loving and open relationships with family and friends
- A sense of community
- Opportunities for full emotional expression
- Play

These are not all the factors necessary to emotional health. But they are some of the most important. We will look briefly at each and consider what we can do to cultivate it.

Self-acceptance: The acceptance and love we receive from other people is an important nourishment for our emotional body. But our love and acceptance of ourselves is necessary for emotional health. If I appreciate and accept myself I am more likely to be a happy person. I will enjoy life more and I will also be more positive in my attitudes and behavior to other people. Some wise person said that the first step to loving life and to loving others is to love oneself. On the other hand, self-rejection is directly linked to depression, antisocial and criminal behavior, alcohol and drug addiction, and other negative patterns.

Accepting and loving oneself is not easy. Probably we are not as attractive, brilliant, talented, successful, and moral as we would like to be. Though we may successfully present a picture of confidence and competence to others, we know the truth about ourselves—that we are at times weak, lazy, incompetent, dumb, and sneaky. Just as "no man is a hero to his valet," neither is any person a hero to himself, assuming that his powers of objective observation are intact. And the person who begins to regard himself as a hero will soon find the universe sneaking up behind him and administering a sobering blow.

For example, several years ago I was traveling through Europe lecturing at Macrobiotic summer camps. I was well received everywhere (or so it seemed to me). I began to think of myself as quite wonderful, a White Knight of Macrobiotics, dispelling ignorance and teaching "the way of life according to the Order of the Universe." The universe did not wait long to disabuse me of this conceit.

I was on my way from Holland to Bern, Switzerland, and on the way visited for a few days in a small town outside Basel. I left some things in a locker in the main railway station in Basel, planning to pick them up later. The train returning to the city was late, however, so I had only four minutes to pick up my luggage and to catch the train to Bern. I was confident though, that as a White Knight, I should have no trouble making the connection. I was wrong.

Before the train halted I leaped off and started running toward the locker. En route, I left my bags at the stairway leading up to the next train. After fetching my things from the locker I began running back across the main hallway of the station. Suddenly, behind me there was a loud explosion. I turned and there on the concrete floor was a mass of shattered glass and foaming, brown liquid. I had been carrying a one-litre bottle of my favorite German beer. This had slipped out of the plastic bag and detonated on the concrete floor. Though dumbstruck, I could see that several hundred dour, stolid, law-abiding Swiss were staring glumly at me, awaiting my next move.

Now Switzerland is probably the cleanest, neatest country in the world. Every night the entire nation is washed and blow-dried. If you are discovered dropping a cigarette butt on the street you are arrested and deported to Italy. So I was confronted with a dilemma: to flee or to stay. The Germanic part of my divided soul told me to stop, pick up the glass, and clean the mess. The American part told me to run like hell and catch my train.

I ran like hell. Cradling the broken bag and its remaining contents to my chest, I grabbed my luggage and sprinted up the stairs to the waiting train. Perspiring and gasping for breath, I leaped aboard with only seconds to spare, and collapsed into a seat. A narrow escape, I thought gratefully. The train, however, did not move. And then persisted in not moving. I started to worry, then to panic. The police had delayed it, I surmised, in

order to arrest me. I expected at any moment a phalanx of
Swiss gendarmes to march up the stairs and take me into cus-
tody. For a moment, nearly overcome with fear, I considered
hiding in the toilet at the end of the car. Just then I noticed that
the train on the next track was departing. Its destination placard
read "Bern." My train was also about to depart—but for Paris.

The incident ended well. I got off the train in time, returned
to clean up the mess I had left, and caught the next train to Bern.
The point of the story is that, in a few short minutes, I went
from being (in my mind at least) a brilliant lecturer on the order
of the universe to a sweaty and terrified fugitive sitting on the
wrong train and contemplating concealment in a toilet. I had
been reminded that behind the cool, competent, and exemplary
person whom I present to the world lurks an incompetent boob.
All of us have such an alter-ego, and if we start to forget that
fact, the universe obligingly reminds us of it.

In the present day, self-acceptance may be particularly difficult.
The media surround us with ideals of youth and beauty, which
make us feel commonplace and old before our time. The traditional, realizable models for the "real man" and the "real
woman" no longer pertain, and have been replaced by impossible
ideals. Women are called upon not just to be nurturing and
loving mothers, but also to be competent mechanics and to have
successful careers. Men are expected to be not only aggressive,
active breadwinners, but efficient housekeepers and tender child-
care supervisors as well. Besides, the world has become so complex, particularly in its social, political, and technological aspects,
that it is difficult, nearly impossible, to understand. One feels
ignorant, powerless, and overwhelmed.

And for the Macrobiotic person there is the added challenge
of adhering to a diet which is not easy to follow. To be a good
and worthy person not only must he be kind and honest in his
social interactions, he must in his eating patterns be consistent,
moderate, and disciplined.

In spite of these obstacles we must learn to accept and to love
ourselves. Otherwise, our chance for emotional health (happiness)

is small. Fortunately there are some simple, practical things we can do to cultivate self-acceptance and self-love. These include the following six strategies:

1. Always keep in mind Schinkhorn's Law. "Given a reasonable opportunity, we human beings will screw up."

Baron Ulrich von Schinkhorn was an Austrian nobleman of the eighteenth century. One day the good Baron was having lunch with his wife, Lady Hulga, on the balcony of their Alpine villa. The Baron was wearing a brand new pair of *Lederhosen* (leather shorts) and a clean white shirt. Suddenly a knockwurst covered with mustard slithered off the baron's plate, rolled down his chest and landed on his lap. Shirt and Lederhosen were well decorated with mustard and grease. The Baron, a Stoic at heart, turned calmly to his wife, and said: "My dear Hulga, it is part of the human condition to screw up whenever the opportunity presents itself." He then emphasized his point by launching another knockwurst from his plate, this time onto Lady Hulga's bright pink dress.

The point of Schinkhorn's Law is that inevitably we make mistakes. We do things that are clumsy, incompetent, and immoral. We should try to avoid them. We should believe and assure ourselves that we will be dexterous, suave, and loving. When we do slip up, we need not be surprised or outraged. We need not hate ourselves, or feel that we are bad or without worth. If we were perfect we wouldn't be in the world at all. We would be floating around on a cloud, strumming a harp with the other angels. Our errors and failings are in fact necessary to our evolution as human beings. This idea brings us to our second strategy.

2. Make every "stumbling block" a "stepping stone." Use every mistake and failure as an opportunity for learning and change.

Behind every blunder and misdeed is a pattern of thought and/or behavior which needs to be changed. If we can objectify ourselves, isolate that pattern, and start to change it, our failures become the impetus for our development into better human beings. Behind my Basel experience was a tendency to schedule my life too fully, with no margins, and thus to be constantly running from place to place. After it, I resolved (for about the fiftieth time) to give myself more time between obligations, and to relax and rest more. Behind the Baron's encounter with the knockwurst was his lamentable tendency to smear too much mustard on sausages and to eat too fast. In its wake, he decided to eat more slowly and to wear a blue nylon jump suit during meals. Every catastrophe, small and large, has something to teach us. It can be an occasion for increasing our skill, under-standing, and virtue. And it can lead to greater self-acceptance and respect rather than to less.

3. Avoid feelings of guilt by dealing openly with misdeeds. When appropriate, confess errors, apologize for them, and make amends.

Guilt is the feeling of unworthiness which results from break-ing a moral law or failing to live up to some ideal. It is perhaps the greatest enemy of self-respect, self-acceptance, and emo-tional health. Many of our problems and sufferings, emotional but also physical, are rooted in feelings of guilt. Thus, it is crucial that we have a way of dealing with guilt before it festers, grows, and demoralizes us.

Many of our blunders are "victim-less crimes." They do not substantially injure or inconvenience anyone except perhaps ourselves. Locking my car keys in the car for the second time in a day, losing my wallet, getting lost on the way home from a party, may be careless and stupid acts, but they injure no one and should not give rise to guilt.

But many of the things we do directly affect others. I drape my wet bath towel over my mother's antique wooden chair. I wake my neighbor by playing the stereo at three o'clock in the morning. I "forget" to pay back a loan from a friend. As with "non-victim" deeds, we need to accept and to learn from these mistakes. But we need also to deal with them in a more active way, lest they give rise to a debilitating feeling of guilt. We need to openly acknowledge these acts, and apologize and make amends for them.

The ritual of confession, apology, and penance is usually associated with courts of law and with churches. But it need not be. It can be used anywhere and anytime and with anyone whom we have wronged deliberately or even accidentally. Even in the most mundane circumstances it is a sacred ritual because it cleanses our heart, releases us from our guilt, and heals our relationship with other human beings.

Once I was leading a panel discussion in front of a large public audience. A woman in the audience kept taking the floor and making what I felt to be irrelevant and self-serving comments. Without an excess of tact I asked her to be quiet for a while. She looked very hurt and angry but was silent for the rest of the meeting.

I soon realized though that I had treated her in an insulting and demeaning manner. I felt very badly about it. I sought her out after the meeting and asked to speak to her. Obviously still upset, she wasn't anxious to do so, but I insisted. I told her I was aware I had spoken to her very impolitely and had embarrassed her in front of the audience. I said I was very sorry, and hoped she would forgive me. Suddenly her face lit up into a smile and she gave me a forgiving hug. Immediately I felt much better and we parted friends.

This was a minor incident. The remorse and guilt I felt was not great and probably would have been soon forgotten. Still I was very glad I acknowledged my insensitivity and apologized for it. The same healing gesture can serve us in more serious circumstances as well, when we have lied, deceived, stolen, broken our word, or been unfaithful. To acknowledge and to apologize for our lapses is not easy. It threatens our sense of self-worth to openly acknowledge a mistake. But since it unburdens us of guilt (and reconciles us to others) it is essential to our self-acceptance and to our emotional health.

4. Remember that food choices are not matters of morality, that therefore "bingeing" is a "non-victim" crime and should not engender guilt.

This is especially important for Macrobiotic people and others trying to follow some food discipline. From a broad perspective, what we choose to eat does have moral implications. If, for example, I buy and consume chicken, I am supporting the chicken industry which incarcerates and badly treats millions of animals. But for the most part, eating is a morally neutral act. We should not feel guilty about some dietary indiscretion though it may seem ill-advised and self-indulgent.

Bingeing can result from any of several factors. Often it is caused by an imbalance in the diet. We may be eating too much Yang food, such as salt, fish and overcooked grains, and therefore are drawn to extreme Yin foods, such as fruit, sweets and alcohol. It may be caused by a nostalgic longing for a favorite treat of times past—vanilla ice cream with chocolate "jimmies" perhaps. Or bingeing can be caused by an extreme and stressful life-style, which makes us tense and leads us periodically to break through all restraints.

Whatever its cause, bingeing should not occasion self-recrimination and guilt. We have not hurt anyone else, and if we approach bingeing positively, we can avoid harming even ourselves. This requires that we observe quality and quantity in the process. Whatever we decide to eat and drink, we should get the best quality available. Also, we should endeavor to consume a reasonable rather than a gargantuan quantity. Thus, if I have a craving for ice cream I can get the best possible honey-sweetened variety. And I can limit my quantity. The best way to do this is to have "participating witnesses"—friends I have invited over to share the feast. The bad effect of bingeing largely comes from poor-quality food eaten in quantity. It comes also from the guilt which we feel after devouring a gallon of ice cream while hiding in our clothes closet.

Even if we binge imprudently we need not feel guilty. We can look on it as an educational experience. One summer day I found myself in a supermarket and, much to my surprise, at the

checkout counter with a very large bag of pretzels and a six-pack
of beer. As I sat outside enjoying my booty, a Macrobiotic
friend came by (they often do at such moments). He looked
at me as if I were mugging a little old lady. "Hi," I said, "I am
performing a scientific experiment to determine the effects of
beer and pretzels in ninety-five degree heat. A breathless world
anxiously awaits the result of my research."

My friend then bought his own bag of pretzels and six-pack.
We ate and drank, talking about the Red Sox, enjoying the
sunshine, and our hour of blissful dissipation.

Occasionally we have to forgive others for what they do to us.
And occasionally we have to ask others to forgive us. Certainly
then we can forgive ourselves for an occasional indiscretion.

5. Periodically make a list of your virtues and accomplishments.

All of us have virtues and strengths as well as weaknesses. All
of us have accomplishments and successes as well as failures.
Sometimes we may forget this positive side of ourselves, and we
can remind ourselves of it. There is a simple exercise called "They
Can't Take From You the Dancing You Have Done." I saw it
first played at an old-age home in New Hampshire.

One of the residents, a lady around eight-five years old was
very depressed. Sound of mind, but very infirm, she was complaining to the nurse that she was worthless, that she was unable
to do anything anymore, even enjoy herself. "Why Minnie,"
the nurse protested, "you are a good and strong woman. You
have had a long life, have accomplished many things, and made
many people happy. Let's play a game to prove it. I want you
to think back over your life, and tell me about all the things you
accomplished from the time you were a little girl. And I will
make a list of them."

It turned out that the old woman was a remarkable person
and had had a rich and rewarding life. She had helped her
parents run a farm in northern Vermont and yet managed to get
a college education. She had been happily married for sixty years,
and had raised five children, all of whom were happy and successful. She had written a book of poetry and was respected in

the home as a compassionate and intelligent person. The nurse wrote down each item as it emerged from their talk, and there was soon a long list. Within an hour Minnie was smiling broadly. She kept that list in her drawer from then on and often, I am told, added to it.

There are times when each of us can bear to be reminded of our achievements and of our measure of goodness. We are all mixtures of Yin and Yang.

6. Periodically study, learn, and master something which does not come easy.

Each of us is naturally skilled at certain things and not so skilled at others. We realize this early in life and generally spend time doing what we do well and avoiding what we do poorly. Thus a child good at drawing and painting and poor at sports will spend much time at the easel and little, if any, on the playing fields. As we get older this tendency to specialize continues. We develop skills in a few areas, but consider the challenges of many areas of life beyond our competence. A woman may, for example, occupy herself principally as a homemaker and feel quite confident and happy functioning in that role. But she may consider fixing a bicycle, making a speech, or going on a camping trip as impossible challenges. Mastering a skill outside her normal range of activities will increase her sense of power and self-worth, and make her a more confident and happier person.

This is the aim of the "inappropriate challenge strategy." It involves choosing a skill, which one would like to learn but for which one feels no aptitude, and then applying oneself to it until some level of mastery is attained.

For example, a friend of mine—a young woman—is very active and athletic. She particularly loves bicycling. Since childhood, she has always owned a bicycle and has used it as her main means of transportation. However, she always considered herself an incompetent when it came to mechanics. So whenever anything went wrong with her bicycle—if the gears got out of adjustment or if she had a flat—she had to take it to the bicycle shop. This was inconvenient and expensive.

Finally she decided to take things literally into her own hands. She began to learn how to maintain and repair a bicycle. She bought several books on bicycle mechanics and repair—classics such as *Bicycle Repair for Dummies*. She read them through and bought the tools recommended. Then she took a course on bicycle repair at the local "Y." She started to attempt small repairs, then larger ones. By the end of a year she could take her entire bicycle apart and, better yet, put it back together. This was a modest accomplishment perhaps, when viewed dispassionately, but for my friend it was a major triumph. She acquired a new expanded sense of her power and potential.

Another example of successfully using this strategy concerns a case of "naturephobia"—the unreasonable fear of nature and the outdoors. A young man, who had grown up in New York City and who prided himself on being an urban sophisticate, decided to get over his naturephobia. He had never slept outdoors in his life and was terrified of the prospect. Nevertheless, he enrolled in a wilderness survival course, struggled through, then re-enrolled. On the third try he completely mastered the course, and so impressed the instructor that he was hired as an apprentice. In time he became an accomplished outdoorsman.

For each of us there are some things we would like to learn or achieve, but which seem beyond us. It may be something as mundane as changing the oil in the car, or sewing a button on a shirt, or playing "Mary Had a Little Lamb" on the piano. Whatever it is, very likely we can master it with a little hard work. And if we do so, we will feel much better about ourselves.

These six strategies can help us gain self-acceptance.

Fulfillment of Vocation: Another key ingredient in emotional well-being is fulfillment of vocation. It can provide the basis for a happy and satisfying life. Its lack can be a source of frustration and unhappiness.

The term vocation has several meanings. Today it usually refers to an occupation, the trade by which one earns a living. Originally, however, it meant a special mission or destiny in life, ordained by God. Vocation comes from the Latin *vocatio* which means literally a "calling." Thus a priest, nun, or clergyman has a "vocation" or "calling," to lead a life of religious devotion or activity.

But the term can be used in a broader, non-ecclesiastical sense. It can refer to the activity or way of life to which any individual is powerfully drawn and which promises a unique and profound personal fulfillment.

Every person has a vocation. Each of us has a mission to accomplish in life, something which we feel deeply called to pursue and realize. Vocations are as varied as human beings. A person's vocation or "calling" may be to raise a happy and healthy family; to collect and annotate the complete lyric poetry of Henry Ford; to become the best handball player in northern New Jersey; to minister to the poor of the world; or to protect some threatened corner of the natural environment.

Whatever our vocation is, it is important that we discover it, dedicate ourselves to it, and realize it as best we can. However humble, a vocation that is at least in part fulfilled, is the basis for a meaningful and happy life. One of the most radiant and contented persons I have known is the bus driver who brought me home every day from junior high school. Each afternoon exactly at 3:06 he would pull up, a beaming smile on his face. During the whole drive he serenaded us with Irish folk songs. Once I asked him why he sang and he replied simply "Because the sun is out and I enjoy what I'm doing."

On the other hand, a person who has no sense of vocation, or a person who has one but does not pursue it, is bound to be unhappy. Witness the sad and aimless drifter through life, never quite sure where he is supposed to be, and what he is supposed to be doing. Witness also the person who knows what he wants to do but does not do it. However filled with wealth, power, and prestige that person's life may be, he will be frustrated and unhappy. And that frustration will affect negatively each dimension of his being—physical, psychological, and spiritual, as well as emotional.

It is a great privilege to be a human being. Imagine an endless ocean inhabited by a single turtle and with a single leaf floating somewhere on the surface. According to Hindu thought, the chance of our coming into the world as a human being is the same as that of the turtle surfacing on that endless sea and taking that single leaf in its mouth. So, given this great gift of human life, we must use it properly. We must do what we really need and want to do. To spend our life doing what is irrelevant and unsatisfying is both wasteful and sad. As Thoreau said, "To kill time is to injure eternity."

We must, then, discover our vocation and realize it. This is not always easy. But with some dedication of time, energy, and will, it is possible.

Some people from an early age have an exact idea of what they want most to do with their life. They know from age nine that they want to be a dancer or a doctor, that they want to amass a great stamp collection, or to climb Mount Everest. These people are very fortunate.

Most of us early in life lack a clear idea of that mission or way of life which will most fulfill us. We have perhaps only a vague sense of what we really want to do. So, when crucial decisions are made, we are influenced by the hopes and expectations of our family, teachers, and peers. We get on one of the well-established, socially-approved "conveyer belts through life." It may be the physician's conveyer belt or the wife-and-mother conveyer belt. Whatever it is, it is designed to take us from adolescence to the grave, comfortably and conveniently. It keeps us busy and satisfied enough that we do not ask whether we are doing what we really want to be doing—until perhaps it is too late.

Whatever our age and our way of life, it is possible, if we have not yet done so, to discover our vocation. And it is also possible to start to realize it. Not only is it possible, it is absolutely imperative.

The first step is to discover our vocation. This is not so difficult. We need only to look deeply into ourselves, and use our intuition and imagination to unveil the secrets of our own heart. There are various ways to do this, fasting and prayer being one time-honored method. The "Orphan-Lottery Exercise" is a less rigorous approach. This requires space (a quiet place where you will not be disturbed), time (an hour or two), and perhaps a pad and paper. It has two stages.

The first is the "Orphan Fantasy." All of us perform on the stage of life with a Greek chorus at our side. This ensemble consists of our parents, brothers and sisters, spouse, children, and other relatives, as well as our friends and associates. Each time we make a major move this chorus reacts, usually with approval or disapproval. If we decide to go to medical shool it will probably respond with cheers and words of encouragement. If we announce our intention to hitchhike penniless around the world it probably will respond with boos, hisses, and words of warning. Sometimes we change our mind because of our Greek chorus's response. Often though, we anticipate its reactions and decide to do what it will approve. Thus this ensemble of loved ones deeply affects the course of our lives.

The "Orphan Fantasy" requires that you imagine yourself living on an island. The entire "review board" of your life —parents, family, friends—has rented a boat to come and visit you. A storm arises and sinks the boat. All are lost and suddenly, tragically, all the people who really love you and care about what you do, disappear from the face of the earth.

You are deprived of their love and support. But you are deprived also of their comments and influence on your life. You are free to imagine and to do exactly what you want to do, or almost so.

You are only "almost free," because most of us do not have the money to do exactly what we wish, even if we know what it is. Do not worry, though. Just proceed to part two of the exercise—the "Lottery Fantasy." Imagine that you have just won the New York State Lottery and are guaranteed an income of a million dollars a year for the rest of your life.

Thus in two swift strokes of fate you have been relieved of the two principal limitations under which most of us live: the expectations of our loved ones and inadequate funds. For a time you are free, albeit in your imagination only, to do exactly what you want to do. You need not worry about your parents or your spouse disapproving. You need not worry about the financial costs involved. You can do exactly as you wish for as long as you wish, within the bounds of legality of course.

Record whatever images come into your mind. Your aspirations may be sensual or spiritual, selfish or altruistic, small or grand. They may include living on a Caribbean beach with beautiful women and an inexhaustible supply of cocaine, or becoming a monk in Tibet; acquiring the world's finest collection of medieval coins or establishing a refuge for homeless people; having a luxurious home and garden or saving the wilderness from acid rain. When you have written your fantasies down, rank them in order of importance. At the top of the list put that aspiration which calls to you most deeply and powerfully, that seems most indispensable to a meaningful life. Very likely that is your vocation. It is more likely to be spiritual than sensual, altruistic than selfish. But whatever it is, so long as it doesn't involve injury to others, it is valid.

Discovering one's vocation is just the first and less difficult part of the task. The other is to manifest it in the real world. When the Orphan-Lottery Exercise is over, our loved ones are there again with their expectations. And the need to earn a living still exists.

The first obstacle is perhaps the lesser. People who really love us will approve whatever we really want to do. They need only be convinced that it will indeed make us happy.

The second obstacle, the financial and practical one, is more difficult for most people to overcome. A few fortunate souls are born wealthy and are free to pursue their dreams as they wish. A few lucky and/or clever people marry such rich souls and share in this freedom. Unfortunately, the rich tend to marry each other, leaving us poor folk to fend for ourselves.

Another group of fortunates are those whose vocation is also a good livelihood. I have a friend who loves old books and who makes an excellent living as an antiquarian book dealer. On a grander scale is a professional athlete like Larry Bird, the basketball player. Bird no doubt loves what he does. But no doubt he loves it more because he earns about twenty thousand dollars an evening running up and down a court, throwing a ball through a hoop.

For many people, though, their vocation is not a source of income, or at least not a very good source. For these the reasonable pursuit of their true "calling" might require sacrifice and compromise. They may have to be content with a lower income and standard of living than they would otherwise enjoy. They might have to pursue their vocation on a part-time basis. Aspiring novelists have a tradition of living in cold, bare garrets in order to realize their dream. And there are people working in the post office who devote evenings and weekends to woodworking or to meditation.

One school of thought regarding vocation (an optimistic one) maintains that if we really discover our vocation and pursue it wholeheartedly, we need not sacrifice nor compromise. It holds that if we are really doing what God and the universe mean for us to do, our income and needs will be well taken care of. According to this "lilies of the field" approach ("Behold . . . they neither toil nor spin . . . ." Matthew 6: 28), we should devote ourselves fully to our vocation even if it does not promise security or wealth. We will, contrary to prospects, be well provided for. As Jesus taught, "Seek first His kingdom and His righteousness, and all these things shall be yours as well."

In any case, it is imperative that we discover our vocation and as much as possible live in harmony with it. We should spend our lives doing what we enjoy most and do best. It is to our own benefit and to that of everyone else. Fulfillment of vocation is essential to our health and happiness.

Loving and Open Relationships with Family and Friends: If we succeed in accepting and loving ourselves, and in fulfilling our vocation, we have gone a long way toward emotional well-being. We are generating within ourselves strong and positive emotional energy. This nourishes our emotional body and benefits every aspect of our life.

The positive emotion generated within ourselves is not enough however. While we are individuals we are not independent beings. We need emotional nourishment from other human beings. We need the affection, compassion, concern, and love of others as assuredly as we need air to breathe and food to eat. And we need to love as well as to be loved. We need to experience and express affection and concern for others. One can starve from lack of love (and of the opportunity to love) as well as from inadequate nutrition. Elderly people, after losing their spouse, often sicken and die, "of a broken heart." And some people are happily sustained for years through loving and being loved by a treasured pet. Thus, open and loving relationships are essential to our emotional and general health.

The natural context for such relationships is our immediate family. With our parents, brothers and sisters, aunts and uncles, with our spouse, and with our children, we share a strong biological, social, and spiritual bond. It is natural that we turn to them for mutual love and support. Our close friends, those brothers and sisters in spirit, can also be a rich source of emotional nurture.

It is important then that we have deep, loving, and open relationships within our family and friendship circle. If we do not have them there we are unlikely to have them elsewhere. To some degree such relations occur naturally and spontaneously. But they do require certain things: that time be spent together; that during this time real interaction and communication take place; that the relationship extend over a long period; and that there be mechanisms for solving conflicts and problems.

Today these factors are difficult to create and maintain, more difficult perhaps than in earlier times. The pace and distractions of modern life reduce the amount of time families spend together. In many homes both parents work and the children are busy in school and elsewhere outside the home. The family may come together only for an occasional evening meal.

Even when there is time together it does not necessarily involve real communication and interaction. The chief culprit here is television. Thirty years ago the focus of family life was the dining room table where meals were eaten, homework done,

games played, discussions carried on. Today the focus is the
television room where people sit in rows, facing not each other,
but the electronic source of vicarious experience. It is hard to
have a meaningful interaction sitting shoulder to shoulder with
someone and watching "Dynasty."

Also, even when there are good relations with family members,
our geographic mobility limits their depth. In our society, many
people move, move often, and move far. Hence, a person living
in Chicago may have siblings in California, Texas, New York,
and London, and parents in Florida. While thanks to the telephone and to air travel, he may maintain these relationships, he
will find it difficult to deepen them. And this mobility stretches
and often breaks ties of friendship. Each time we move to a different city or region we must create a new circle of friends and
struggle to keep contact with those we left behind.

We may need then, especially within our family circle, to consciously nurture deep and affectionate relationships. This may
involve changes in life-style. We may, for example, have to in-
tentionally spend more time together, making our family a high
priority and ignoring some of the distractions outside the home.
The Mormons, who value family life very highly, observe one
night a week as an inviolable "family night." All members are
present and they do something together. We all may have to
adopt this or a similar practice just to insure that we share
enough hours in a busy week.

We may also have to rediscover old and more intimate ways
of spending time together than watching television. These include
playing games (Scrabble, Parcheesi, charades), doing puzzles,
reading books and stories aloud, putting on plays, performing
music together, holding semiformal discussions on topics of
common interest. All these activities were accepted ways of daily
family amusement only a few decades ago. They brought family
members together in active and enjoyable pursuits. They fostered
deep relationships based on communication and shared experience.

We may need also to learn new ways to deepen individual
relationships. Family interactions, involving several or many

people, usually limit the communication any two people can have. The *tête-à-tête* or intimate one-to-one conversation is a good way to cultivate a deep and satisfying relationship with the individual members of one's family. A friend of mine has a sister who lives several hours distant. He sees her and her family on holidays and other family occasions. But every month he meets her and takes her out to lunch. And he uses the time to really explore what she is feeling, thinking, and doing. He never opens the conversation by asking "How are you?" since it invites the dead-end reply, "Fine, how are you?" Instead he asks a specific question usually beginning with the phrase, "What are you feeling about. . . ." Thus, typical conversational gambits are "What are you feeling about your new job? What are you feeling about Mom having to go to the hospital?" His sister, in fact, has gotten adept at asking the same kind of questions. Their monthly luncheons have helped them to understand and to love each other very deeply.

We may also need to reconsider our national addiction to mobility. Our nomadic life keeps us separated from family and periodically wrenches us from established friendships. Several years ago I was traveling in central Europe. After some weeks in Germany and Austria I noticed a clear difference between the two countries. While in Germany there was a rather grim and frenetic atmosphere, in Austria the general feeling was much more relaxed and peaceful. I asked a friend (an Austrian) about this and he replied, "The main difference between Germany and Austria is that here we consider our family and friendships the most important thing. So if we are offered a better job in another city we usually turn it down. We cannot bear leaving our native place and the people we know and love. In Germany they are more likely to accept it and move. I have turned down several promotions which would have involved moving."

Spending more time with our family, making it meaningful time, and arranging our lives so that close relationships can continue and deepen throughout our lives, are each important in developing the loving relationships that we need. Also important is some way of resolving the conflicts and problems that inevitably occur. Family relationships are seldom easy. The first husband and wife, Adam and Eve, quarreled in the Garden of Eden. And the first siblings, Cain and Abel, also came into conflict. Problems arising from the generation gap between parents and children are almost universal. The positive emotions are very close to the negative ones, and when conflicts arise, concern can easily turn into contempt, affection into anger, and love into hate. It is vital then that we deal with these inevitable conflicts positively and with dispatch.

Many families get professional help in the form of "family counseling," to deal with their conflicts. In some cases this may be necessary. However, it is preferable to deal with family problems without paying someone sixty dollars an hour. And in many cases this is possible. We need to have a technique for exposing and resolving conflicts and to use it when they arise. Conflicts and the emotions they engender—annoyance, resentment, anger—are like mushrooms. They grow best when left undisturbed in the dark. Exposed to the sunshine and fresh air, they tend to shrivel up and disappear.

There are various ways to bring conflicts into the open, to confront them openly and honestly, and to resolve them. One is an exercise called "Appreciation-Confrontation-Suggestion-Agreement (ACSA)." I learned it first twenty years ago from a friend in Chicago. He had just been through a drug rehabilitation program in which ACSA had been used to help the "residents" deal with conflicts. It can be used by groups of various types and sizes.

I have used ACSA with most of the Outward Bound groups I have led over the past fifteen years. On an Outward Bound course, a group of eight to ten people, accompanied by one or two instructors, lives in an outdoor (usually wilderness) situation for a period of six to twenty-six days. Cut off from all other contact, these strangers become a *de facto* family. The wilderness environment, whether it involves hiking, canoeing, or climbing, is usually physically and psychologically stressful. For the first several days things go pretty smoothly "in the family." People are polite, helpful, and friendly. However, usually by the fifth

day a problem has developed. For some reason, some person
(or persons) is angry at some other person (or persons). There
may be no obvious indication of this except a palpable psychological tension in the group. It is crucial though that it be dealt
with before it develops too far. So we play ACSA.

The group sits in a circle so that each person can see the face
of everyone else. Each person in turn becomes the focus of attention. The others are free to give that person positive and negative
feedback. They must do so, however, in a specific manner. First,
they must point out something they like, admire, or respect
about the person. They must express "appreciation" of the
person. Then they may draw attention to something that is
troubling them about "the focusee." It must be something which
that person can control or change—a pattern of behavior for
example, rather than a physical characteristic. Telling someone
that you can't stand the color of his eyes is a dead-end street.
This "confrontation" is followed by a suggestion of what the
focusee can do to eliminate the troublesome situation. This
"suggestion" is followed by a discussion and it is hoped, by
an "agreement" between the parties on some course of action
which will resolve the issue.

For example, on a particular trip there is a fellow from Minnesota. His name is Mike and he shares a tent with Bill. When
Mike is in the "hot seat" (as the focus position is sometimes
called) Bill says:

"Mike, I really appreciate how helpful you have been to me
the past days. You taught me how to put up the tent, how to
stay warm at night, and a lot of other things. BUT (this word
usually is a good indication that the appreciation is over and the
confrontation is at hand) I do wish, that you wouldn't get up
every morning at 5 o'clock and yodel for an hour. I wake up
and can't get back to sleep. So when everyone gets up at 7:00,
I'm still tired. Is there any chance that you could practice yodeling at another time of day?"

Very likely Bill will be quite surprised by this. It never occurred to him that his yodeling was loud enough to disturb
anyone. (Most of the things we do which bother others we are

largely unaware of.) He replies, "I'm sorry Mike. Back in Minnesota everyone yodels in the morning, but I can do it in the afternoon after lunch." Thus, suggestion and agreement have followed appreciation and confrontation and the problem is solved.

As we go around the circle a variety of issues come up, some major, some minor, but all potentially problematic if left untended. Mike, in fact, has a comment for Bill. He says that although he is glad that Bill takes the cooking responsibilities for them both, he would be happier if the breakfast oatmeal did not contain seaweed. Bill, apologizing, agrees to substitute raisins.

By the end of the session, which may go on for hours, several things are clear. One is that most people are uncomfortable with the process, especially at first. We live in a culture where civility and cordiality are more valued than honesty and directness. We are not used to being open about our thoughts and feelings, particularly if they are negative. And we dislike doing it. We are afraid we will hurt other people's feelings, that they may not like us for what we say. Also, we probably do not like getting frank criticism in return.

It is also obvious that the process is very valuable to each individual and to the entire group. Free to speak honestly and openly, each person can express feelings and thoughts which have been causing tension within him. He feels purged, refreshed, relaxed. Also, because the tensions between people have been resolved, the energy flow within the group is much stronger and freer. The group as a whole feels purged, refreshed, and relaxed. ACSA functions as a kind of emotional acupuncture, releasing blockages of energy and restoring a harmonious, healthy energy flow.

"Appreciation-Confrontation-Suggestion-Agreement" can be played by two people or as many as twelve or fifteen. While it works well with groups such as those on Outward Bound, it works equally well with groups who work, study, or live together, with traveling companions, friends, and with members of a family. Used periodically within a family, it can help to resolve problems and conflicts and to bring people close together, in affection and understanding.

Of course not all problems and conflicts can be resolved by ACSA or by any other technique. Sometimes people are unwilling or unable to change their patterns. In such a situation, just getting the issue into the open is very helpful. Then all parties, particularly the aggrieved, must exercise patience, tolerance, and respect so that a single issue does not undermine or destroy a relationship or the group.

Many Macrobiotic people confront just such a problem with their families on the issue of food. Let us say that Mary has become Macrobiotic and has greatly benefited from the diet. She goes home to visit her elderly parents full of missionary zeal. Her father has a heart condition and her mother has asthma, and she is sure a change of diet will help them. Her parents, however, do not want to be helped, at least not by eating brown rice and sea vegetables, and they politely resist her attempts to change the eating habits of a lifetime. Mary coaxes, cajoles, begs, and pleads. She cooks dinners and gives *shiatsu* massages. But all is to no avail. She feels angry, rejected, hurt. And her parents in turn feel pressured and put upon. A lifelong, close, and nurturing relationship is about to founder on the issue of diet.

Having a family is something like having a special, custom-made (by an enemy) hand. This hand is connected to the central nervous system's *afferent* (hand to brain) nerves only. There are no *efferent* (brain to hand) nerves. This means that we experience what happens to this hand but we have no control over what it does. Unfortunately, this hand seems to delight in doing things which give it (and us) discomfort and pain. It puts itself on the hot stove. It sticks itself with pins. We feel this pain very deeply. But when we tell the hand to stop it ignores us. It may in fact redouble its efforts to mutilate itself. We love this hand very much (we cannot help loving it), so in order to stay in relationship with it (not to cut it off), we must be very patient, understanding, tolerant, and respectful.

At some point then, Mary has to accept her parents as they are. She must respect their decisions about what they eat and

how they live. She must love and accept them even though they
will not become what she wants them to be. This will be easier
perhaps if she remembers that her parents love and respect her
not because of what she eats, but in spite of it. Her parents are
probably privately shaking their heads and thinking, "How can
she eat that food? She is killing herself."

The same respect and tolerance is needed if our other relations—our wife or husband, our children or our friends—also
fail to "see the Macrobiotic light." Each person has his own
unique path through life and we must respect it, even though it
may not agree with our own. It is unnecessary and shameful to
injure a relationship because of disagreement about diet.

Creating and maintaining loving relations with our family and
friends is not always easy. It requires time, energy, sacrifice and
the willingness to criticize and to be criticized. It requires tolerance, humility, and respect. But it is an important, necessary
enterprise, well worth our every effort. To be full, healthy, and
happy human beings, we need the love and support only those
closest to us can afford. Without it, we are in danger of starving,
as surely as we would starve without food and drink.

A Sense of Community: Another important ingredient in
emotional health is a sense of "community": the feeling that we
belong to a larger social organism than that formed by ourselves, our family, and our close friends.

A community is a group of individuals who have something
or things in common. Place of residence, occupation, ethnic
background, history and traditions, way of life, religious beliefs,
and a vision of the future are among the things which can be
the basis of community. These factors bind people together,
giving them a sense of common identity and welfare.

Throughout history most human beings have lived in a community, formed by several or many of these common factors. In
medieval Europe, for example, most people were born and lived
their whole lives in a village of perhaps a hundred people. These
people lived close together. They all made their living by farming,
or some related trade. They came from the same ethnic stock

and shared a common history as well as blood. Their food, clothing, homes, furnishings, language, and patterns of behavior were all the same. Most or all had the same religious beliefs, the same view of the universe, and expressed these regularly together in church. The village then was a community tightly bound by many common factors and each person was an integral part of it.

Even today some people live in strongly-knit, clear communities. In rural areas this is still the dominant pattern. And in urban areas as well, many people live in "ethnic" communities, held together by a common neighborhood, national background, way of life, and religion.

From life in such a tightly bound, coherent social organism, one derives a "sense of community." It includes a clear idea of who and what one is, and of where one's place is. It includes as well a sense of worth in the world, since one shares in the stature and accomplishments of the community. It includes a sense of security, since one knows that in case of personal and familial difficulties, others will come to one's aid. It includes too a sense of strength and importance, since in times of need, one will be called to help others. This "sense of community" is important, perhaps essential, to our emotional happiness.

Some people in modern society, however, belong to no single, strong community. The typical city dweller or suburbanite is part of several separate, unrelated social groups. These are bound by only one or two factors and thus are not true "communities." Thus he lives in a particular neighborhood but shares little other than space with his neighbors. He works in a company, but does not socialize with his fellow workers after hours. He goes to church but sees his fellow parishioners only for that hour or two a week. Shuttling between these several "one-dimensional communities" he feels no strong attachment to any of them. Thus he lacks a "sense of community" and the feeling of identity, of self-worth, and of security which it gives. He suffers to some degree from the disease of *anomie*, or the sense of rootlessness, aimlessness, and alienation, of having no place, purpose, or identity in the world. According to the French sociologist, Emile Durkheim (1858–1917), anomie is almost unique to modern urban humanity.

Many of us today, therefore, have to work at finding a community and developing a sense of community. There are various ways to approach the problem. Twenty years ago young people began to experiment with communal living, and the commune movement blossomed on the American social landscape. This was an attempt to create intentional communities of like-minded persons, usually in a rural setting. Some of these communities have succeeded and survived. Many have not. In the more individualistic decade of the eighties, the idea has gone a bit out of fashion. But the possibility is still there and the communal alternative may again come into vogue. It is also possible by moving to a small city or town to regain this sense of community.

For those unwilling or unable to live communally, or to move to a small town, the challenge seems great. Our cities are vast, impersonal, and overwhelming. The "communities" in which we function are fragile and one-dimensional, held together by common place, occupation, ethnic background, political views, or religious beliefs, rather than by a combination of these. Nevertheless we can develop a nourishing community involvement. We need only to be aware of our situation and to deal with it consciously and creatively.

Involvement in a church, neighborhood, company, or other "one-dimensional" association can provide a satisfying sense of community. What is important is not the type of community but our commitment to it and our active involvement in it. A community is a family and friendship circle writ large. Like a family, it requires time and energy, self-sacrifice, ability to resolve conflicts, as well as tolerance and understanding. We may live in an immense, impersonal metropolis. But we can consciously and energetically involve ourselves in a small part of it, in a church or religious group, a neighborhood association, professional group, or school. If we do so, we need not suffer from anomie. We can be emotionally nurtured by the sense of identity, security, and power which community provides.

I know a woman who lived alone for years in New York City. An artist, she had a small circle of friends but knew almost no one outside it. She felt very lonely and isolated. One evening at a dinner party she met another women and they fell into conversation. Soon they realized that they lived in the same part of Manhattan, on the same street, in the same building, and even on contiguous floors. They had in fact been living within fifty yards of each other for six years and had never even seen each other. The artist said to herself (with some insight), "This is crazy!"

The next week she went around to all the apartments on five floors of the apartment building, introduced herself and told her fellow tenants (almost all total strangers to her) that she was forming a "neighborhood association." In time, after some hard work, she got the thing going. It developed into a thriving "mini-community" with monthly potlucks, occasional outings, and picnics. Even in New York, it is possible to satisfy the tribal instinct when the will is there.

For people involved in a spiritual discipline or path, such as Yoga, meditation, or Macrobiotics, making others with the same interest the "community of focus" can be very rewarding. Associating with those who share our aspirations is enjoyable and interesting. But also it is helpful to our own striving. A synergy or combining of energies takes place, and the will, skill, and achievement of all is increased.

When a person enters the Buddhist monastic order three vows are taken: "I take refuge in the Buddha. I take refuge in the Dharma (the teachings of the Buddha). I take refuge in the Sangha (the community of monks and nuns)." Gautama the Buddha established the order and the vows knowing that it is much easier for a person to follow a spiritual path, or any other discipline, if he is surrounded by and helped by others sharing his path and goal.

We human beings are social creatures. We need to be part of a community, a social unit that transcends the family. We need to feel accepted, recognized, important, and secure. We need also the opportunity to help and protect others. This tribal instinct is very deep and persists even in the heart of modern urban humanity. Our fulfillment of it, even in the context of a segmented and atomized society, is crucial to our emotional health and to our general well-being. Thus, cultivating a community involvement and developing a true "sense of community" is a vital part of the Macrobiotic way of life.

Opportunities for Full Emotional Expression: It is important that we express our emotions, the mild and positive ones, but also and particularly, the powerful and negative ones. Anger, fear, resentment, frustration, and grief involve energy which if not released can affect the entire organism in a significant and devastating way.

Repression of emotion is a problem especially for people from northern European backgrounds. In Scandinavia, Great Britain, and in the Germanic countries (also Japan), there exists a tradition of emotional reticence. To openly express a feeling, positive or negative, mild or intense, is considered undignified and unseemly. Emotions are to be held and hidden. Thus the typical Swede, if his bride happens to burn the toast on the wedding morning, harbors his resentment for the next thirty years. During that time it (along with all the other repressed negative affects) creates an emotional tension that permeates the person's body, mind and spirit.

In southern Europe, among the Greeks, Italians, and Spaniards, repression is less of a problem. These peoples are uninhibited about expressing their emotions. If they are angry they shout, stamp, and gesticulate until they are no longer angry. I was on a bus in Greece once, and every few miles the driver flew into a violent rage at some person or object on the road. I was beginning to question his sanity and to fear for my safety when my neighbor (a Britisher who knew the country) explained that this was "business as usual." Similarly, the Latin people are more expressive of their positive feelings of affection and approval. The hearty embrace is part of social life all through the Mediterranean, among men and women. In Stockholm it is a cause for uneasiness. The expressive approach to our emotions, while making daily life more dramatic, also may be conducive to good health.

Whatever our ethnic background, we need to express and

release our emotions. This is true even of positive emotions. Much pleasure, joy, and positive energy is lost to the world by the unnecessary repression of good feeling. A gratuitous smile, a whoop and a holler, a spontaneous hug of affection and appreciation, each sheds a bit of emotional sunlight, warming to all. The repression of good feeling is the waste of a valuable resource.

Dealing successfully with negative emotions is crucial. Each of us, inevitably, at times feels grief, anger, fear, envy, remorse. At that point we can do either of two things. We can express the emotion fully. Or we may repress it. For example, at the death of a friend we may cry and beat the ground until the grief starts to subside. Or embarrassed about our feelings, we can keep them within us. Emotions if fully expressed have no further claim on us. Repressed emotions stay with us and exert a negative influence until they are released. They can issue in emotional problems such as chronic depression. They can also contribute to difficulties in our other bodies. Excess muscle tension and decreased organ function, stifled artistic creativity, and antisocial behavior patterns, can all have a basis in repressed emotion.

It is important then that we learn to express rather than repress emotions. This does not mean that every time we feel angry, or fearful, we need to enact a public drama. Many negative emotions can be released very subtly.

For example, suppose I am waiting in line at the bank and someone pushes rudely in front of me. I have several options. They are, in increasing order of intensity, as follows:

- I can take ten deep, slow breaths. I can tell myself that this person may have a good reason to be in such a hurry— perhaps his pregnant wife, about to give birth, is waiting in the car. I can look at the situation in perspective and realize that, after all, I am being delayed only a few moments, that there is nothing worth getting upset about. I can thus reduce or eliminate my emotional response so it ceases to be a problem. Such a strategy works best in trivial circumstances. In more serious ones it is difficult and can easily lead to an undesirable repression of feeling.

- I can use a version of ACSA, mixing up a little Yin and Yang, sweetness and reprimand. I might, for example, very calmly tap the man on the shoulder and say: "Sir, I imagine you are in a hurry, but it bothers me that you cut in. Perhaps you could go to the end of the line." This is confrontational of course, and if the fellow happens to be six-foot-six, I must be prepared to beat a hasty retreat.
- I can address him a bit more heatedly, saying "You dirty S.O.B.! Get to the back of the line. You think you're Princess Di or somebody?" This is more expressive but increases the risks a bit too.
- I can try without a word to drop him with one punch. However satisfying this may be at the moment, it is probably an unnecessary escalation of the conflict. Besides, it is applicable only if the opponent is short and frail. Also, with opponents over sixty years of age, or on crutches, this is generally not considered good form.

Whatever option I choose, I should avoid standing there and stewing in my own emotional juices. The same is true when the words or actions of family members, friends, or associates really bother us. Probably some version of ACSA in this and other circumstances is the most desirable option. It is a perfect combination of Yin and Yang, compliment and reprimand, stroke and sting, expression and control. Used with consideration and compassion, it can help us avoid the ill effects of bottling our emotions.

A confidant, a person who is compassionate and trustworthy, and who will listen to us speak our heart and mind, is very helpful in dealing with our emotions. There are anxieties, fears, regrets, sorrows, and angers as well as joys and aspirations which we may choose not to express in public or even among family and friends. Thus a person to whom we can reveal in confidence all our feelings and thoughts is a great blessing.

Anyone can fill the role of a confidant. It can be a brother or sister, a member of the clergy, an old and trusted friend. Today some people are so estranged from family, friends, and from the religious establishment, that they have no one to whom they can vent their heart. They have no one who will listen to them without interruption even for an hour. These people often wind up in the offices of counselors and psychiatrists. They simply need someone who will listen to them patiently, with concern and without judgment.

Some years ago a movement called "Peer Co-Counseling" began in the United States. It is based on two ideas:

- We all do need someone to whom we can reveal all our emotions, thoughts, and concerns.
- Almost anyone can be trained to be a skilled confidant and counselor.

Individuals interested in the program take a course of about ten sessions. They learn to listen "creatively," that is, attentively, using questions and comments to bring out the real feelings and thoughts of the speaker. After the course the members pair off and make an agreement to meet regularly. In the sessions each person talks about his problems and emotions for a specific time (an hour or so) with the other person as creative listener. Thus each person is confessor and confidant, patient and counselor. These relationships sometimes continue for years, and are of great help to those involved.

Even without the training, a pair of friends can benefit from the insights of this program. They might meet regularly, and agree that each in turn has an hour to speak about his own concerns. The listener has to be attentive and, except for questions and comments no longer than one sentence, silent.

Sometimes of course the emotions which trouble us are ones of which we are scarcely aware. They may be related to childhood or even infant experiences. They may originate in experiences so traumatic that we cannot consciously confront them.

In these situations, some professional aid is advisable. Both conventional psychiatry and "alternative" approaches can be helpful. The latter include a wide variety of techniques involving counseling, body work, or both. Rolfing, Primal Scream Therapy, Rebirthing, and Gestalt Therapy each claim many practitioners and many people have been helped by them. These therapies can be an excellent complement to the Macrobiotic diet and the Macrobiotic way of life.

Play: Children at play are marvelous to behold. Absorbed in their own space, time, and amusements, they are oblivious to past and future and to the world around them. We adults watch them with a mixture of awe, nostalgia, and envy. We recall how, without the cares of job, family, and the world upon us, we too easily slipped into the special world of play. That world for us now probably seems distant and inaccessible.

If so, it is unfortunate. While we human beings refer to ourselves as *homo sapiens* ("man the wise") and *homo faber* ("man the maker of tools") we are also, perhaps pre-eminently, *homo ludens* ("man the player"). Play is natural to human beings at every stage of life. While we may play less as we grow older, that is perhaps not the result of old age, but the cause. It is not that we do not play because we are old, but that we are old because we do not play. Throughout our life, we need play. We need those moments when, lost in play, we transcend space and time, and are uplifted and refreshed by the subtlest energies of the universe. Play is essential to our health and happiness.

What is play? It is a pastime that is active, amusing, absorbing, aimless, and harmless.

Play is active in that it requires the movement of the body and/or the mind. Running can be play. Playing chess or watching the changes in the sky can be play. Sleep or its waking counterpart, watching television, are not play.

Play is amusing in that it is pleasant and fun. However, it need not at every moment be enjoyable. Play can involve challenges and difficulties that are at times downright unpleasant.

Thus mountain climbing, and rigorous competitive sports, can be play. Hanging by one's thumbs is not generally considered play.

Play is absorbing in that it causes one to lose awareness of time and space, and even of one's self. If we are truly at play then nothing can easily lure us away. Children enjoying their games in the early evening are often reluctant to heed the call to dinner.

Play ideally has no other justification than itself. As such it is aimless. It is pursued not for profit or any other end. Certain types of play do produce results. The play of professional athletes earns them a living. But it is still play in a pure sense if the participants would take part regardless of the rewards.

Play is harmless in that it causes no injury to oneself or others. Thus war, taking drugs, hunting animals "for sport" are not play. Stalking animals with a camera is play.

Thus a wide range of activities can be considered play, from football to chess, from housebuilding to bicycling around the world. If we cultivate a "playful attitude," everything we do can be play. George Ohsawa said that the truly healthy and happy person is always at play, from the moment of waking to the moment of falling asleep. Play and happiness are the twin sides of a coin, each a cause and a result of the other.

If we have lost the habit and the ability of play, we must regain it. First we must discover an activity that for us is true play, is active, aimless, amusing, absorbing, and harmless. This may be quite hard, since our society is based on activities which are either passive or profitable. But play can be very simple. It can be watching the birds in the sky, or bouncing a ball against a wall. It can be a hobby, or a sport.

Once we have our form of play, we need to indulge ourselves in it till it becomes truly absorbing, till it makes us smile and laugh. Laughter is a sure indication of true play. It is the tonic of rejuvenation and the surest medicine for all ills. A person who is always smiling and laughing, who is always at play, is a truly Macrobiotic person, regardless of what he eats.

Self-acceptance, fulfillment of vocation, loving and open relationships with family and friends, a sense of community, full expression of our emotions, and play are all important factors in our emotional life. There are of course many others. But our conscious and energetic cultivation of these few will provide a firm basis for the health of our emotional "body" and for our entire self.

5. Mind Does Matter

Happy the man who can search out the causes of
things.
                                    Virgil (70–19 B.C.)

Health and intellect are the two blessings of life.
                                    Menander (c. 342–292 B.C.)

In addition to our physical, aesthetic, and emotional "bodies,"
we human beings have an intellectual "body," or mind. The
mind deals with realities more ethereal than sense impressions
and emotions, with images, thoughts, and ideas.

The human intellect is a marvelous tool, with varied capa-
bilities. These include observation, memorization, analysis, induc-
tion, deduction, comprehension, and imagination. The mind
can collect information about phenomena in the world (largely
through the sense organs), classify it, and record it in memory.
The mind can analyze this data, discerning recurrent patterns,
and relationships of cause and effect. It can formulate principles
and universal laws based on this data. The mind can use these
principles in specific circumstances to explain, predict, and control phenomena. And it can combine information and ideas in
new and original ways to solve problems and even to invent and
create new phenomena. The human intellect is a wonder indeed.
Its active use, along with our extensive reliance on the credit
card, distinguishes us from most other creatures in nature.

For example, sometime in the immemorial past one of our
ancestors met a friend who was sitting on a log which was lying
across another log. When our ancestor sat down on the far end
of the log his friend was thrown a few feet in the air. Another
day, walking in the forest he stepped on a thick branch which
was balanced on a rock. The other end of the branch flew up
and struck him with unsuspected force. After a few similar
experiences he realized that a long object resting on a balance

point can, if pressed at one end, generate a great deal of force at the other. He discovered the principle of the lever. He began to apply this principle to various situations. He moved large rocks by prying them with a pole. He broke thick branches by jamming one end between two trees and pushing on the other end. Other people learned this principle and applied it, and over generations it issued in a wide variety of inventions from the wheelbarrow to the mechanical clock.

We human beings use our intellectual abilities not only because they allow us to function in the world. We use them because their exercise is pleasing to us. We have a natural curiosity regarding the world. We want to know about and to understand the vast, complex, and fascinating universe in which we live, including its plants and animals, rivers and mountains, microbes and galaxies. We are curious also about ourselves and other human beings. We want to understand what we are and how we function. We want to know what has been thought, spoken, and done in the past, and what is being thought, said, and done now. Each of us is by nature a scientist, historian, and journalist.

The active use of the mind, of its ability to collect and retain data, to discern patterns, to generalize, to predict, to explain, to solve problems, and to imagine and create, is essential to our health and well-being. An active mind is a powerful nexus of energy in the human organism. It stimulates and strengthens each of our other "bodies." On the other hand, a stagnant mind, one whose natural curiosity and many abilities have been allowed to atrophy, negatively affects every other dimension of our humanity.

In the first decades of life the human intellect is very active. The world is full of new stimuli and information, of an endless torrent of things to be observed, discovered, analyzed, remembered, understood, and comprehended. And the healthy child is always wide-eyed with curiosity, and with discovery.

Most of this activity occurs in normal day-to-day life. Just in being alive and aware, in going through the day observing the world, other people, and himself, the child or adolescent acquires knowledge, formulates general truths, and applies them to

specific situations. Intellectual activity in early life occurs also
in schools. A primary aim of formal education is to stimulate,
nourish, and train the mind. Methods of gaining information,
of thinking, and of problem-solving, are taught and practiced.
Study of the world is pursued in a clear systematic manner. The
object of study is explicit and the methods of study orderly and
precise. One focuses on grammar, mathematics, history, biology,
on some discreet aspect of the natural or human world. In
schools, colleges, and universities, the level of intellectual activity
is usually high.

For many people, once they pass out of childhood and young
adulthood, vigorous intellectual activity radically decreases. For
some it virtually disappears. The spontaneous discovery and
learning of the fresh and growing mind slackens. Formal education ends. Some discovery, problem solving, and learning
continue—in meeting the challenges of family life, in doing
one's job, in observing and reading about the world. But
usually this is random, unfocused, and without rigor. After
graduation from high school, or college, most people, unless
they are professionals or intellectuals, go into intellectual eclipse.
Even the very bright and the highly educated experience this.

There are various factors behind this common abdication of
the life of the mind:

- Formal schooling, despite its good intentions, can be too
  intense, stressful, coercive, or dull. It leaves people with
  a negative attitude toward learning, and a resolve never to
  tax their intellect again, unless absolutely necessary.
- We are dominated by the idea that education is the special
  domain of the young, and that the continuing life of the
  mind is the special domain of "intellectuals," such as teachers, professors, and writers.
- We are opiated by a massive media network, including
  television, radio, and the press, mainly concerned that we
  are enough entertained to tolerate their "commercial mes-
  sages." These advertisements may encourage us to buy a new
  deodorant or automobile, but they seldom urge us to under-

take the study of Elizabethan poetry, or to do research on the migratory habits of Canadian geese.
- There seem to be few resources and opportunities for continuing to develop the mind.
- We are (let us face it) lazy.

Whatever its reasons, the decline of intellectual life is tragic and unnecessary. It is tragic because, for three-quarters of our life, we deprive ourselves of one of its chief joys and satisfactions. To think clearly, to solve problems, to use our imagination are among the real pleasures of life. And to acquire knowledge and understanding of the world also is a great joy. Disciplined and focused learning is exciting and rewarding, a "banquet of the mind." It can be, as well, a means to personal and even spiritual development. It broadens us and deepens our connection with the rest of creation.

Each intellectual discipline focuses on an aspect of the natural or human world. The natural sciences look at the world of nature; the applied sciences and technology at the machines and processes of the human-made world; the social sciences at human society and psychology; history at the past; art and literature at the creations of human aesthetic genius. Each branch of study allows us to comprehend one particular dimension of the world. "Comprehend" literally means to take something into one's hand, to grasp, that is, to make part of oneself. Thus by study we can incorporate something of the world into ourselves. We can expand the bounds of our ego, become broader and richer, more related to the world.

For example, if I go into the forest with no knowledge of trees, I will see many cylindrical and leafy forms. I may find them aesthetically interesting, but generally they mean little to me. If I have studied *dendrology* ("the science of trees"), however, I can look at and experience each tree, knowing its type, its age, its past and future, and its patterns of growth. I am surrounded by familiar forms, by friends and fellow living organisms, whom I know about and understand. I can comprehend the trees and forest, take them into myself and become larger through it.

Similarly, we make ourselves larger by our knowledge of the plays of Euripides, by our understanding of the operation of a computer, by our acquaintance with Freud's theory of the human psyche.

The atrophy of intellectual life is unnecessary because the life of the mind can continue throughout life. While our physical abilities decline with age, most of our intellectual powers remain the same or even increase. It is true, that while we are young we can absorb information and concepts (especially in mathematics, abstract science, and in the study of foreign languages) more quickly and easily than when we are older. But our powers of observation, reasoning, imagination, and problem solving develop and increase with age. Plus, we bring to all our studies our experience of life and of the world. Thus, especially in the humanities, such as literature, history, philosophy, and psychology, our ability to understand and comprehend improves with age. Plato and Confucius, two great minds who graced the earth in different places but at roughly the same time (fifth century B.C.), shared an interesting opinion about age and study. Both said that the study of philosophy (the most basic issues concerning the universe and human life) can only begin at age forty, and that it must continue till death.

Thus our "education" need not and should not end when our formal schooling ends. In fact it really only begins then. Our formal schooling should have taught us how to use our minds and how to learn. As adults we are free to use those abilities exactly how we choose. We can thereby enrich our lives until the end of our days.

It is possible and important then that we remain intellectually active throughout our lives. We need not become lifetime students or professional intellectuals. We must however continually exercise our intellectual abilities. We must take in information, analyze and absorb it. We must keep our problem-solving and imaginative abilities alive and sharp. In other words, we have to nourish and exercise our intellectual body just as we must nourish and exercise our physical body. The many ways to do this include the following:

Read Selectively, Widely, and More: There is a saying in Zen Buddhism, "Throw away your books." The implication is that reading and the absorption of information and ideas which it involves are a hindrance to spiritual development. But as mentioned, study can enlarge the ego beyond its narrow limits and help us embrace other phenomena. Thus it can be an aid in spiritual striving. That Zen proverb might be rendered, "Throw away your books after you have read them." Mr. Ohsawa, who usually championed intuition over intellect as means to knowledge and personal evolution, was nevertheless a voracious reader who read five or six books a day.

Despite the rise of the electronic media, of TV, radio, and the movies, reading is still an unparalleled way of getting information, ideas, and stimulation. Books and other forms of reading matter are cheap, portable, and available in tremendous variety. For a few dollars we have access to virtually any topic imaginable, from medieval farming to the role of computers in raising livestock. For a trip to the library we can communicate with the great writers and thinkers of human history. Books, magazines, and newspapers are a marvelous resource but we must learn to use them well.

We can, for example, read selectively. The world is awash in print, and more is created every day. We are able to read only a fraction of what there is and of what is continuously being produced. Not all printed matter is equal. Some is trivial, banal, and transitory; some informative, inspiring, and of lasting interest. Some intend only to fill an idle moment. Some seek to inform, instruct, and elevate the mind. There is a difference between the police page of the morning paper and a page of poetry. There is a difference between a novel of trite gothic horrors and Dickens' *David Copperfield*.

We can therefore carefully choose what we read, even as we carefully choose what we eat. Certainly light, diversionary, and current reading matter has a place in our lives. But what is informative, inspirational, and classic, should occupy perhaps a greater place. We can read newspapers and magazines choosing informative and substantial pieces and passing over those which record the endless calvalcade of human folly, violence and catastrophe. In selecting books we can choose a masterpiece by Shakespeare, Hardy, Plato or Rabelais rather than the latest, soon to be forgotten "best seller." As the English philosopher Ruskin observed "Life being very short and the quiet hours of it few, we ought to waste none of them reading valueless books." A truly "great" book provides timeless wisdom as well as pleasant diversion.

In our serious reading we can read widely, that is, in a variety of areas: in history, the natural sciences, the social sciences, literature, economics and politics. We might even do so with some plan so that we give some attention to each of these "liberal arts." The *ars liberales*, "the arts of the free man," comprise that broad body of knowledge which distinguishes the free citizen from the "slave." Today it is possible to graduate from a respectable "liberal arts" college and be totally ignorant of vast areas of human knowledge. (I know—I did it!) So it is up to us to broaden a narrow and specialized perspective, and to make ourselves into liberally educated persons.

Most people have little time to read. But it is possible to increase one's reading even without increasing the time actually spent sitting at home, book in hand. Even in the busiest life there are spaces, moments of waiting or of inactivity. We spend minutes, often many minutes, waiting in doctor's offices, or in line at the bank, post office, and supermarket. A paperback book, always kept handy, can turn these minutes into enjoyable, useful ones. The alternatives are limited. In a check-out line we can contemplate the chewing gum and cigarette displays or read the frontpage article of the *National Enquirer*, pieces like "Baptist Preacher Explodes During Sermon." We may be better off with a book of short stories by Chekhov.

Many of us spend a lot of time driving, often alone. Commuting time can be a relaxing lacuna in a hectic day, but it can easily get boring, after about seven minutes. Fortunately, there are companies that produce, rent, and sell books recorded on cassette tapes. Some offer hundreds of "books," classic and contemporary fiction, biographies, mysteries, and even "how-to" and self-improvement books. "Literature," of course, originally was something recited and listened to, rather than printed and read. Listening to a good novel can be a remarkably enjoyable and powerful experience. I used to dread long, solitary drives but now, equipped with a recorded book, almost look forward to them.

Consider Everyone a Teacher: Our daily social contacts offer opportunities to increase our knowledge and understanding of the world. Every person is a walking encyclopedia of information and wisdom. So, each person we meet—at a party, on an airplane or bus—young or old, rich or poor, attractive or ugly, knows many things we do not know. And in most cases he is happy to share that with us. On a trip back from Europe once, I sat next to a young woman who worked for a mutual fund investment corporation in Boston. A nosy journalist at heart, I asked her question after question. She was pleased with my interest and in a few hours increased my knowledge and understanding of the financial world about a hundredfold. And in the exchange she learned a lot about bicycle travel. Even the most wretched derelict sitting on a street curb could, if we took the time to really talk with him, teach us much. The world is full of teachers, and most of them are not in classrooms.

Take Advantage of the Electronic Media as an Educational Resource: Television, radio, and the movies aim to entertain first and to educate second. And that educational motivation is usually a distant second. Still, there are many programs and movies which are informative and intellectually stimulating. The national public television and radio networks, in particular, daily present (with no commercial interruptions) interesting and worthwhile offerings on current events, nature, history, literature, and art. The commercial networks also have valuable programs, but with enough advertisements to addle the mind in the process. Taking advantage of these offerings involves a sacrifice. A program on sixteenth century religious art may come head-to-head with "Miami Vice," or "Three's Company." The need to choose between pap and real nourishment appears here as it does in every area of life. We need entertainment and relaxation as well as education. But we need them in balance, and today the scale is tilted to the first two.

Always Ask "How?:   Every day we use materials, products, and devices about which we may know little or nothing. We may have no clear idea, for example, how plastic is produced or how it is formed into the myriad products which surround us. We may have little understanding of the principles, let alone the particulars, of the operation of our radio, television, or personal computer. "Kotzsch's Double Law of Applied Ignorance" pertains to this unfortunate situation. It says, "Never use any material or product without knowing how it is made. Never use any machine without knowing how it works." We needn't acquire detailed and expert knowledge, but we should have a general idea of the processes and mechanisms in question.

Adhering to the "Double Law" is no mean feat. It requires at the minimum, some good reference books at home—at the least, an encyclopedia, atlas, dictionary, and almanac. These will be useful in following the next suggestion as well.

Always Ask "Why?":   Every phenomena we experience poses a question: "why?" Why is that street named Baker Street. Why does that man have red hair and dark circles under his eyes? Why does dried fruit taste sweeter when it is cooked? Why did the Europeans colonize the world beginning in the sixteenth century. Why? Why? Why? We can keep our intellectual faculty sharp by answering this question as often as possible, regarding the minutiae of life as well as the grand issues.

People who have studied Macrobiotics and the philosophy of Yin and Yang have two excellent tools for understanding phenomena. These are the law of the alternation of opposites and the understanding of the role food plays in human life. These are useful in looking at any issue. Often they afford insights which academic-scientific explanations do not provide.

For example, we can apply these tools to the history of

European colonialism. Beginning in the sixteenth century, people from a geographically insignificant part of the world (Europe is really just a tiny finger sticking out of Eurasia) went over the world and subdued much of it. Why did they try it? Why did they have the strength and fortitude to accomplish it?

The climate of northern Europe is cold, damp, and dark—very Yin. The plants, animals, and human beings which survive and flourish there must of necessity be very Yang. Rendered Yang by the demands of the climate and eating its Yang foods—meat, eggs, salty cheese, baked breads—the inhabitants became extremely Yang. Physically active and strong, they ultimately reached the Yang extreme. Restless and aggressive, feeling confined in their native lands, they set out in search of an opposite environment (a warm, Yang, easy one) and of opposite foods (sweet, succulent, stimulating, Yin ones). They went all over the earth, but mainly to the tropical and subtropical areas in Africa, India, China, and South America. They conquered the milder and less technically advanced (more Yin) people there. They appropriated and brought home the various Yin delicacies to which they were attracted: sugar, coffee, spices, tea, cocoa, and opiates. According to the laws of Yin and Yang, everything is attracted to its opposite, and eventually changes into its opposite. Thus, after some generations of enjoying these Yin foods, the imperial nations became physically and mentally weak (Yin), and were unable to hold onto their empires. The colonial period ended.

Mr. Ohsawa constantly urged his students to analyze and understand every phenomena, keeping in mind Yin and Yang and the hidden but important role of food.

Become an Expert on Something: Systematic, thorough, and extended study of one subject nourishes and exercises the intellect in a unique way. Each particular phenomenon is a microcosm of the universe, and contains the complexity and unity of the cosmos itself. Thus, the in-depth study of one person, one country, one period of history, even one battle in one war, a single novel, mountain, or animal can be an endlessly instructive and rewarding project.

Many people, neither writers nor professors, but homemakers, business people, and workers, have as an enduring, even lifelong hobby, the deep study of one thing which has caught and held their interest. They study the Battle of Gettysburg, a species of butterfly, the history of lace making in America, or the maintenance and repair of old watches. There is an international organization called "The Baker Street Irregulars" whose members study the life and work of Sherlock Holmes. Any serious and continuing study helps keep the intellect alive and well.

Use Games to Keep the Mind Active, and the Memory and Problem-solving Ability Alive: Chess, bridge, Scrabble, "twenty questions," charades, crossword puzzles, riddles, and other recreational activities, exercise and stimulate the mind. They are like a workout routine for the intellect, keeping it from getting flabby.

Throw Away Your Calculator: The mind is like any muscle. If it is used it gets strong. If unused, it atrophies. Mathematical calculation is an exercise which keeps the mind strong and flexible. The electronic calculator is fast and accurate. But for every advantage there is a disadvantage, wherever there is Yang there is Yin. So, as the use of the calculator increases, the mental ability of the user decreases. I have a very bright friend who has used a calculator so long that without it he can barely subtract five from ten. Some people rely on these machines for their livelihood, but most of us use them as a debilitating crutch.

Exercise Your Memory: From time immemorial the human memory has been used to record information. The invention of writing, then of moveable type, and more recently of electronic memory, have step-by-step reduced its importance. So today most of us use our memory for little more than finding our way out the front door. But the human memory is still a marvelous and important tool. I have a friend (ironically enough the same fellow who is addicted to his calculator) who memorizes poetry. He knows by rote several hundred poems and at any moment can recite the many stanzas of Wordsworth's "Tintern Abbey" or Coleridge's "Rime of the Ancient Mariner."

Learning a poem, or passage from a book by heart is a good way to strengthen and tone our intellectual faculty. It is also a way to internalize beautiful and inspiring material. Until recently, it was an important element in public and religious education.

Use Opportunities for Continuing Education: To help round out our "liberal education," to answer particular questions of "how" and "why," to pursue a special topic of interest, to stimulate our problem-solving ability, and to exercise our memory we can use the resources of formal education. There are many opportunities for formal and disciplined study for adults. Evening schools, YMCA's and YWCA's, community colleges, college and university extension programs, and adult-education centers all offer inexpensive courses on a myriad of subjects. Enjoying the guidance of an instructor as well as the stimulus of other students, one can nourish and exercise the intellectual "body." These opportunities exist in every community, town, and city. They need only to be sought out.

These are just some of the many ways we can nourish and exercise our minds. They involve resisting some of the lures of contemporary mass culture. They require therefore a clear intention and an energetic, consistent effort. But they issue in something crucial to our overall health and well-being, a vital and full intellectual life.

While most people today suffer from a lack of intellectual exercise, some suffer from an excess. These include students, teachers, lawyers, writers, accountants, computer programmers, and others whose primary activity is intellectual in nature. And here again too much of a good thing can be as disruptive as too little. The human organism thrives when there is a balance between the activities of its various "bodies."

Excessive intellectual activity can negatively affect the mind itself. It can reduce curiosity, the pleasure taken in learning, the power of memory, and the acuteness of the reasoning abilities. But mental overwork can influence the physical, emotional, and other areas of life as well. It can lead, for example, to low physical energy, muscular tension, emotional depression, and to a lack of interest in personal and social relationships (sometimes referred to as the "Nerd Syndrome").

Such symptoms indicate a serious imbalance. A person suffering from them should reduce the time and energy spent in intellectual pursuits. And he should increase that spent in physical exercise and in aesthetically and emotionally satisfying pursuits. It is natural that many of the people involved in jogging, bicycling, and other aspects of the fitness movement are students, intellectuals, and professionals who may overwork their intellectual "body."

The human mind, then, has the ability to observe, analyze, and comprehend the world and the phenomena in it. To be full and healthy human beings we must throughout our lives exercise and develop this ability. But the mind can also influence and shape reality, our own and that of the world around us. If we understand this fact and use it wisely, we can greatly improve the quality of our lives.

Everyday thousands of images, ideas, and concepts pass through our minds. Each is a unit of energy with a particular quality and strength. Each affects our mental state, but each affects as well our entire organism. Our thoughts influence how we feel physically and emotionally, how we speak and how we act. And they influence how others respond to and act toward us. Our thoughts may also affect the material world of inanimate objects. Matter is compacted energy and thoughts are more diffuse, faster-moving energy. Some people claim to move or bend objects *telekinetically*, by the power of thought alone.

From a holistic or monistic view of reality this is certainly possible. Each of us may be affecting the material world around us all the time without being aware of it.

While we have a great many distinct thoughts in a day, we have relatively few different thoughts. We have a limited repertoire of images, ideas, and concepts which keep repeating in our minds over and over. Because each of these "mental habits" is played many times each day, it has a major affect on us, on the people and the world around us.

Mental images and thoughts may be positive or negative. Negative thoughts are unpleasant and pessimistic. They are dominated by images of disorder, violence, ugliness, pain, decay, and death. "Life's a bitch and then you die," is a common and unmistakable negative thought.

Negative thoughts create negative realities. A negative mental image creates an energy field which influences the person who thinks it, and external objects and other people as well. Thus, as studies indicate, pessimistic and self-demeaning persons have a higher than normal incidence of cancer. People who dislike or distrust machines often are given reason to do so. I have a friend who dislikes wearing a watch. However expensive a timepiece she buys, inevitably it stops working within a month. And people who expect failure, often do fail. Suppose that I am asking my boss for a raise. I am not convinced that I deserve it though, and expect to be turned down. My negative attitude causes me to speak without confidence or conviction. Its negative energy field engulfs and influences my boss as well. Very likely I will be turned down. This is an example of the "self-fulfilling prophecy," a mental image which helps to manifest itself. A sick person who does not expect to get better probably will not recover.

There are many varieties of negative concepts which we play on endless looped tapes in our little mental tape player. Some are very specific and individual ("I have a funny looking nose so no one will like me."); others are more general ("Today is going to be filled with unutterable catastrophes."). Many of them, however, are versions of one of the following, general, insidious negative mental attitudes:

- "I am a helpless victim of chance and circumstance."
- "If I try something new and difficult I will fail."
- "When I fail at something it means I am no good."
- "Every difficulty is to be avoided at all costs."
- "If anything can go wrong it will."
- "Life has given me a raw deal."

Positive thoughts are pleasant and optimistic. They include images of growth, efficacy, power, harmony, peace, and beauty. "Life is good and worth living," and "Today will be full of excitement and fun," are positive ideas.

A positive image and thought helps create positive realities. It generates a positive energy field which affects the thinker himself. A sick person given a neutral substance (*placebo*) but told that it is an effective medication, may be as likely to get well as someone who actually has received the medication. Similarly, a person with cancer who focuses on images of health and wholeness, of the healing forces in his body removing the cancer cells, may help his recovery. This visualization technique is helpful in areas other than therapy. It may, for example, improve athletic performance. A high-jumper who actively visualizes himself clearing the bar at a record height increases his chances of doing so.

Positive images and expectations can affect objects and other people as well. My friend has a 1961 Chevrolet, and is absolutely convinced it will "run forever." The car has just passed the 250,000 mile mark! The self-fulfilling prophecy works with positive expectations as well as negative ones. If I drive downtown convinced I will not find a parking place, probably I will have difficulty finding one.

Positive thoughts, like negative ones, can be specific and personal ("In spite of the rain and the crowds I will immediately get a taxi.") or general ("All weather is beautiful weather."). Like negative thoughts, most are a variation of one of several major themes. The following are important positive concepts. We have already encountered some, as expressions of the Macrobiotic world view.

"I am responsible for everything that happens to me."

This idea affirms that I have created myself and my life and that I have power over the future. It opens the door to positive and intended change. It counteracts the victim mentality, and all the anger, resentment, and fatalism which that creates.

"What I sincerely believe I can do, I can do."

The accomplishment of any goal depends on the belief that it can be accomplished. If I am confident of doing something, the energy of the expectation will help me succeed. A "fire-walk experience" I had in New York several years ago graphically demonstrates this point. The leader was Anthony Robbins and for five hours he worked to convince us that the seemingly impossible was indeed possible—if we believed it so. Then at midnight four hundred people each walked over a twelve-foot bed of glowing coals. Such an experience shows that we are limited by fear and self-doubt as much as by reality; and that sincere belief in ourselves liberates us to accomplish almost anything.

"The only failure is to stop trying."

Failure is an intrinsic part of the human experience, whether we are trying to become a morally good person or to solve a difficult problem. As Robbins pointed out in his seminar, Thomas Edison had 500 "unsuccessful" experiments, while developing the incandescent light bulb. In every enterprise, as long as we learn from each attempt and momentary setback, and do not cease trying, we cannot fail.

"What doesn't kill me makes me strong."

While difficulties are in the moment unpleasant, they always have a "back" or paradoxical good side. Yin and Yang always go together. Cold, hunger, poverty, and all other hardships temper and strengthen us as the swordsmith's fire tempers the new steel. A poor and difficult childhood often produces a re-sourceful and remarkable adult (Joan of Arc, Benjamin Franklin,

Charles Dickens). And a period of trial and suffering in later
life can lead to a new insight or achievement. In a conflict
between people from a difficult environment and people from
an easy one, the former usually trimph. For millennia in China
"barbarians" from the cold and arid north periodically attacked
and conquered the developed "civilization" in the temperate
south. The Great Wall was built to keep them out. Thus when
we meet difficulties we should rejoice and be thankful for them.
In fact, in our present-day society of convenience and ease, we
should perhaps actively seek out difficulties and challenges.

"The universe supports my good intentions without reservation."
If we expect things to work in our favor, if we anticipate help
and good fortune, they will come to us. If we accept "Murphy's
Law" ("What can go wrong will go wrong.") we help create
a world in which this is true.

"Life is a blessing and we can never say 'thank you' enough."
Our very existence is a marvelous gift. Even in the worst of
circumstances there are more things to be thankful for than to
regret. And the difficulties which plague us may in the end turn
out to be blessings. Mr. Ohsawa said that the truly Macrobiotic
person is saying "Thank You," constantly and equally for everything—blessings and difficulties, sunshine and rain, life and death.

Our mental habits, those images and thoughts running constantly through our mind, are very important. They deeply affect
the quality of our whole life. As the following brief tales demonstrate, a single thought, positive or negative, can incline a person
to contentment and happiness or to resentment and dissatisfaction.
There were once twin boys, sons of a royal family. They were
equal in strength, character, and ability. When the boys were
about twelve, their father the king grew concerned about which
would succeed him. To avoid later competition he decided that
the boys would draw lots. The winner would in time become

king. The other would be sent immediately to another country. The lots were drawn, the future monarch chosen and the other lad dispatched to a foreign land.

In his new home this second boy was apprenticed to a wealthy merchant and given every advantage, comfort, and privilege. In time he married the merchant's daughter, amassed great wealth through the business, and had several fine children. But this man could never forget his origin. He could never forget that but for the choosing of the false lot he would have been a powerful king.

So throughout his life he was obsessed by the idea that he had been victimized and deprived. His every experience was colored by the recurring thought, "If I were only king. . . ."

Thus when he beheld his wife, who was a lovely and devoted woman, he would think, "If I were only king, I would have ten such as these and all more beautiful than she." And when he contemplated his riches he would reflect, "If I were only king I would have a thousand times as much money, plus land and men-at-arms." And when his sons grew to manhood and entered his business and shared his wealth, the man thought, "If I were only king, my son would follow me to the throne."

So this merchant, once son to a king, led a privileged but very unhappy life. He had all the blessings of life, in greater measure than most other people. But he was dissatisfied, regretful, ever plagued by the mental refrain, "If I were only king. . . ."

In that same period, in that same land, a son was born into a very poor family. Both parents died when he was young, and left on his own, the boy got involved with a band of thieves. Eventually he was caught stealing horses, and was tried, judged guilty, and condemned to die. The day before the hanging, however, twin sons were born to the royal family, and the king in a gesture of celebration pardoned the horse thief. The young man was given a few coins and sent into the town.

He wasn't given exactly a hero's welcome, but he managed to survive digging ditches, running errands, and doing other menial work. Ostracized by the citizens, he lived alone, with neither wife nor family. But this man was quite content, even happy. Always in the back of his mind was playing the refrain, "Thank God I wasn't hanged." However backbreaking his labor, however long the nights of solitude, he always thought, "Thank God I wasn't hanged." And so he was able to appreciate and enjoy even his meagre lot.

It is very important then that we have positive rather than negative tapes in those tiny tape players in our heads. We can achieve this in various ways. One is to keep each of our other "bodies" healthy. Our physical, aesthetic, and emotional condition each affects our thought and mental attitudes. Thus, if I am physically exhausted or hungover from drinking, my thoughts and mental set will reflect that. And similarly, listening to a Mozart symphony or having a violent argument with a friend will also affect my thoughts. Thus, part of cultivating a positive mental attitude is the creation of a positive, healthy state in each part of our lives. We need to eat properly, exercise, express ourselves artistically, and nurture our emotional needs. We need also, as will be discussed presently, to cultivate a healthy moral, ideological, and spiritual life.

But the mind is affected also by its own nourishment, the images and ideas which it takes in, and by the way it handles that "food." We can help develop a positive mental attitude at the intellectual level itself.

We can for example monitor our mental food, go on an "intellectual diet." Our thoughts and patterns of thinking are in large part determined by the images and ideas which we take in from other people, from newspapers and books, from movies and television programs. Friends who are constant complainers, eternal critics, or prophets of doom, literature which focuses on the bizarre and seedy side of life, and movies and television programs filled with gratuitous violence all predispose us to negativity. And optimistic and wholesome people, books, and programs impart their positive quality to the images and thoughts in our mind.

Many cultures have appreciated this fact, particularly in relation to pregnant women. In Japan, for example, pregnant women are advised to avoid any person, event, environment, book, and entertainment which is negative, violent, or perverse. This practice of *taikyo* or "prenatal education" is believed to protect the mental, and also the physical and emotional health of the mother and child.

Each of us is "pregnant," creating by our life today the person we will be tomorrow and next year. So, a like caution is advisable. We need not, we obviously cannot, avoid all experience of negativity. Pain, suffering, violence, and death are part of reality and necessary to it. But we need not dwell on them. I know a person who is a "news junkie." From the moment he arises to the minute he goes to sleep he is reading newspapers and news magazines, listening to news on the radio, and watching it on the television. He feeds his mind a steady diet of crime, murder, corruption, and war. And his mental state reflects this. He is very critical and pessimistic, always dwelling on the faults of others and on the problems in the world. A week watching Laurel and Hardy shorts and Walt Disney features might benefit him greatly.

Also, we can examine our habits of mind and try to change them. The human mind, marvel that it is, can observe itself thinking and can change itself. Most of us have particular negative tapes that we run over and over in our mind. We can recognize them, and learn to replace them with their positive antidote. For example, I may have a well-worn "victim" tape playing in my mind. It repeats endlessly, "I have been messed up by my family and my education," and locks me into a state of resentment and inactivity. Every time I hear that tape playing though, I am free to eject it and put in the positive antidote.

Affirmations can help us replace negative ideas and thought patterns with positive ones. An affirmation is a simple, forceful expression of a positive, optimistic, inspiring idea. "Today is going to be a wonderful day" is an example of an affirmation. "I am responsible for my life and everything in it" is an antidote affirmation for the "I am a victim" thought pattern. It can be repeated aloud fifty or hundred times or until the negative thought

disappears. An affirmation repeated fifty times, several times
a day, mentally or aloud, or written out over and over in long-
hand, or pasted on the bathroom mirror, can imprint itself on
our mind and displace deeply imbedded negative thought
patterns.

There are available today a variety of courses aimed at personal transformation and development. These include the Dale
Carnegie Courses, the Silva Method of Mind Development, and
The Course in Miracles. While they vary in particulars, all are
concerned with changing negative thought patterns, which inhibit and injure us, into positive patterns which liberate and
give us power. While it is possible to monitor and to change
mental habits by oneself, it can be very difficult. Such courses
then can be very helpful.

Thus maintaining a vital and rich intellectual life, and developing positive habits of mind are essential to the health of the
mind. And crucial then to our overall health, they are an intrinsic part of the Macrobiotic way of life.

6. Life is with Others

Morality is not properly the doctrine of how we
make ourselves happy, but how we make ourselves
worthy of happiness.

Immanuel Kant (1724–1804)

Although we human beings are individual organisms, we seldom
if ever function as individuals. We are by nature social creatures.
We enjoy the company of other human beings. Most of us
choose to be with other people every day throughout our lives.
Periods of isolation are rare and brief. On an Outward Bound
course, students have a "solo" experience in which they are
alone for a period of one to three days. For most, this is their
first experience of real solitude, and while they find it valuable,
they are usually quite glad when it is over.

Every day we interact with a wide variety of individuals. Some
we know very well, some a little, some not at all. And we interact with them in a variety of situations, intimate or impersonal,
momentary or protracted. Thus, on a single day we breakfast
with our spouse and children in the morning; we sit next to a
total stranger on the commuter train; we have a conference with
our boss at work; we speak on the phone to a customer in California; we buy stamps from a clerk at the post office; and we
enjoy a leisurely dinner with an old college friend. With each
person and in each situation we must decide what to say and
what to do.

These decisions are very important. What we say and what
we do profoundly affects others. It also profoundly affects us.
Our behavior towards others creates what can be called our
social or moral "body." Like each dimension of ourself, this
moral body is connected to every other body. It is affected by
and affects our physical, emotional, and other dimensions. If a
person tells a lie, even a "white lie," various important changes
occur in his physical condition. Pulse and respiration rate, and

electrical conductivity of the skin change immediately. On his emotional body a gleep of guilt is created. (A "gleep" is an international unit for measuring guilt, developed by the Lutheran Church of America, and is equal to the amount of moral regret generated by cheating on a federal income-tax return.) Thus every act, moral and immoral, affects the moral body and each other aspect of our being. And our moral life is a crucial factor in our health and happiness.

Every culture has wrestled with the question of what it means to be a "good person," to act in a way which issues in the well-being of others and of oneself. And each culture, in its customs, etiquette, and ethical ideals has expressed its view of "moral goodness." These have varied to some extent. In some cultures it is permissible to have one wife, in others to have three or four. In some cultures it is permissible to kill and to eat animals, in others it is wrong even to harm an insect.

Despite this diversity in particulars, one recurring theme runs through the moral teachings of all cultures, past and present, East and West, North and South. It is found in virtually all the religions of the world. This is the Law of Reciprocity. It suggests that we should act as we would have others act.

The Law of Reciprocity can be expressed negatively. In the *Analects*, Confucius declares, "Do not do unto others what you would not have them do unto you." The Hindu doctrine of *ahimsa* or "non-injury," which forbids causing pain or injury to any other creature, is also negative in expression. Thus, as we do not like to be demeaned, exploited, lied to, cheated, stolen from, attacked, injured, or murdered, we should not demean, exploit, lie to, cheat, steal from, attack, injure, or murder others.

The Law of Reciprocity can also be expressed positively as in the familiar Biblical injunctions, "Do unto others as you would have them do unto you," and "Love your neighbor as yourself." Thus, as we like to be treated with honesty, respect, kindness, compassion, and love, we should treat others with these very things.

There is a difference between the two expressions. The first emphasizes avoiding injury to others. The second emphasizes actively supporting, protecting, and nurturing others. In actual practice, though, they amount to much the same thing. Mahatma Gandhi, who took the principle of ahimsa as the central principle of his life, understood it to be identical to Jesus' "Law of Love."

With the Principle of Reciprocity as a yardstick, it is easy in most situations to judge what is the moral course. We need only put ourselves in the place of the other person and imagine how we would prefer to be treated. Some situations involve moral dilemmas. Suppose, for example, that my friend has committed a crime, and the police ask me for his whereabouts. If I lie and say I do not know where he is, my friend will benefit and the police will be thwarted. If I tell the truth, the result will be opposite. Both alternatives involve benefit and injury and it is hard to say which is the moral and which the immoral act.

In most situations, however, the moral and immoral options are very clear. For example, if a distant relative drops in unexpectedly, I can refuse him at the door, explaining that I am sorry but I am leaving for Antarctica in a few minutes and I haven't begun to pack yet. Or I can put aside what I am doing, invite him in with a smile, and treat him with all the hospitality I can muster. Clearly, the second course of action is the loving and moral one. There is no real dilemma here, except perhaps between my own convenience and the well-being of my relation. And this is no true dilemma. The law of love suggests that where the claim is a reasonable one, we put the interest of the other person above our own.

In our effort to be a "good person" we must keep in mind a number of things. One is that while actions must follow the Law of Reciprocity, thoughts and words must do so also. What we think and say as well as what we do can be moral or immoral.

Let us suppose for example (going back to our yodeling vignette of Chapter 4) that I am in Bill's position. Every day I am being woken up by my Wisconsin tentmate. Despite our "agreement" Mike serenades me into wakefulness one cold, rainy morning. I awake, startled and angry. I grab my flashlight and try to insert it forcibly into Mike's wide-open mouth. I knock him over and open a cut on his lip. While my act may be emotionally understandable, it is still a violation of the Law of Reciprocity. I have obviously injured Mike. I have not treated him with kindness.

I may forego violence, and instead just yell loudly at the yodeler. "Mike, you dirty S.O.B.," I scream, "You have done it again. I wish you would go out and play blindfolded on the top of a cliff."

In this case, while I have not struck Mike, I have still done him violence and injured him. When we speak we are creating vibrations in the air. These vibrations vary according to the loudness of our voice, the emotion behind the words, and the meaning of the words themselves. A shout can have a palpable physical impact. An angry voice carries the violent energy of the anger. And words expressing anger intensify that violent effect. Thus words have weight, have power, and they can affect a person very profoundly. An angry tirade such as my outburst against Mike is really an act of violence. Though more subtle than a physical blow, it still injures Mike. His nervous system, his aura or energy field, his emotional body have all been deeply affected. He feels ashamed, hurt, perhaps physically exhausted. These affects may last longer than the pain caused by a blow to the mouth.

Waking to Mike's yodeling, I may choose to do and say nothing. I just lie there tired but awake, stewing in anger, and thinking negative thoughts about Mike. I imagine him being interrupted in mid-yodel by a raging she-bear. I wish upon him a terminal case of laryngitis.

The violence in this case is yet more subtle, but it is equally real. My angry thoughts form a black cloud of negative energy which, directed toward Mike, slowly but effectively engulfs him. He may suddenly feel uncomfortable, anxious, even depressed. Again the effect may last a long time.

Thus to avoid hurting others we must carefully consider our words and thoughts as well as our actions. Abusive language, profanity, malicious gossip, nagging and constant criticism, even a pattern of complaining are immoral in that they create negative energy which affects others. A comment as apparently innocent as "Gee, Harry, you look tired today" can be immoral in that it harms another. Harry, who has been feeling fine until that moment, will be ashamed that he looks tired, and may even begin to feel tired. Likewise, negative and antagonistic thoughts about other people are immoral. If I wish that someone fail in a project or suffer some misfortune, I am injuring them as surely as if I had struck them.

Because they do have weight and power, words and thoughts can be used positively as well, to nurture, support, and aid others. A sincere compliment, a word of encouragement, an expression of appreciation and gratitude, even a comment pointing out the positive aspects in a difficult situation are all moral and loving gestures. Each creates and transmits positive energy. Thus, if I comment on the excellent job my employee has done on a difficult project, I have done a good deed. If, marching through a mosquito infested forest, I draw my friend's attention to the beauty of the spring flowers, I have likewise in a small way obeyed the Law of Love.

Thoughts too can be a powerful force for good. To think of a person in a positive way, to imagine them well, happy, and content is to contribute to that reality. Idea precedes and produces manifestation.

The Law of Reciprocity pertains in every social interaction, even in brief and unimportant encounters with strangers or people we scarcely know. I may, in getting on the bus, salute the driver with a cheery "Good morning, sir," or I may just grumble past, throwing my money indifferently in the box. I may, in leaving my bank, compliment the manager on her efficient handling of my problem, or ignore her. In each case, the impact of my behavior is radically different. Such choices seem as much a matter of etiquette as of morality. But etiquette consists of social forms designed to make others feel respected and important. And thus its observation can be an expression of concern and love. Almost from moment to moment in our lives we have the choice of creating positive or negative energy.

Interactions with institutions are as important morally as are interactions with individuals. Suppose that a mistake has been made in my favor in my bank statement. A deposit of $60.00 was recorded as one of $6,000.00. It is very tempting to just accept the good fortune. The bank after all is an institution, and a large, rich one at that. But institutions, however large and impersonal, are in fact made up of individual human beings. The bank includes the person who made the error and also the bank owners who will lose through my gain. To fail to report the error would be a subtle, but real violation of the principle of ahimsa. It would be the same as stealing from a family member, friend, or any other individual.

Even our relations with the great majority of humanity with whom we have no direct contact are subject to the Law of Reciprocity. The Law of Love suggests that our compassion and help should go out to anyone suffering or in need. In the parable of "The Good Samaritan," Jesus indicates that the truly moral person is willing to succor a person unknown to him. These are the unfortunates in our own society and around the world. They may be in temporary or chronic need. They may be suffering from hunger, disease, poverty, or simply loneliness. They include the homeless derelict surviving an urban winter, the old woman abandoned in a state rest home, and the wealthy suburbanite couple in despair over their health. Each of us, through material and financial contributions, social activism, volunteer work, and through promoting and teaching Macrobiotics can help people with whom we have little or no direct contact. Humanity, like the universe itself, is an integrated organism. The fortune and suffering of each person is related to that of each other person. Perhaps, as Herbert Spencer (1820–1903) said, ". . . no one can be perfectly happy until all are happy."

Even our treatment of ourselves involves moral choice. Each of us is free to take good care of ourselves or to abuse ourselves. We can eat a wholesome diet, get plenty of exercise and fresh air. Or we can gorge ourselves on rich foods, drink and smoke heavily, and otherwise dissipate ourselves. We tend to think of such decisions as matters of personal preference. Even if we use cocaine or marijuana, we probably consider this a

personal matter, at worst a "victimless" crime and thus not really
a matter of morality.

But actually our care of ourselves is a matter of morality.
Dissipation is not evil in itself. But it does affect us negatively.
It undermines our health and happiness. And we do not live in
a vacuum. Our condition and circumstances affect the members
of our family, our friends, our employers. A tree in the forest
seems to be an independent organism. However, because of the
intertwining of roots beneath the ground, it is intimately connected to all the other trees. When one tree sickens and dies
all are affected. They are in fact a single organism. In the same
way our health or sickness affect those around us and society
as a whole. We need not, as noted earlier, become guilt-ridden
about indulging ourselves on occasion. But we should keep in
mind that caring properly for ourselves benefits those around us
as well as ourselves.

Thus our thoughts, words, and deeds, in relation to people
close to us, but also in relation to strangers, to institutions, to
people whom we never see, and to ourselves, are all important
in forming our moral body. But we live also in relation to animals, plants, and to the earth itself. And vis-à-vis these phenomena also, we must abide by the Law of Reciprocity.

We human beings comprise a very small minority of the
creatures on the earth. There are billions and billions of insects,
reptiles, fish, birds, and other mammals who share the planet.
We treat these creatures in various, often contradictory ways.
Some, such as cats and dogs, we take into our homes. We feed
and protect them and lavish affections upon them as pets. We
grieve when they die and perhaps even erect a monument to
their memory. Other animals such as cows, goats, and sheep,
we domesticate, but primarily for their food and economic value.
We take good care of them but deprive them of their milk or
eggs or warm coats. When it suits us, we kill them for their meat
and hides. Other animals we use in scientific research. We test
new drugs, cosmetics, or medical theories on them. Often this
research causes the animals great suffering. Recently, eight monkeys whose spinal cords had been severed for the sake of science

were put to death "for humanitarian reasons." We treat animals
in nature with a similar confusing (to them perhaps, if not to us)
inconsistency. Some fish and game we pursue and take for food.
Bear and other big game we hunt primarily for the "sport."
Yet others (the rat, mouse, and mole) we exterminate as pests.
Some, such as the whooping crane, when they approach extinc-
tion we treat like priceless treasures. Upon most other creatures
in nature we lavish relative indifference.

The Principle of Reciprocity pertains, however, in our relations with all animals. We cannot know exactly how animals
experience life. But several things are evident. They, like us,
feel pain and they prefer to avoid it. They prefer life to death
and will struggle against their own destruction. And, the higher
animals, at least, respond to care and affection. In the most
basic experiences of life, animals, particularly our fellow mammals, differ from us more in degree perhaps than in kind.

Our treatment of the other creatures on the earth, then, is a
moral issue. The Law of Reciprocity applies to it as it applies
to our treatment of other human beings. The "good" human
being does not pointlessly injure, exploit, or kill an animal. A
good human being treats animals with respect and kindness.

Most of us do not abuse the animals with whom we come in
contact. We care for our pets. If we keep chickens and goats,
we treat them decently. We probably do not hunt simply for
blood lust. We do not perform cruel experiments on mice or
monkeys in our basement. We may swat an occasional fly or
trap a troublesome mouse, but we do this more in self-defense
than cruelty.

Indirectly however we may be supporting the wanton and
cruel treatment of animals. Every year, four billion chickens are
killed in the United States alone. These are not chickens who
have had a gay and carefree life in Farmer Jones' yard, pecking
and clucking happily, and trysting behind the henhouse with the
rooster. These are pitiful creatures which have spent their entire
life in a tiny metal cage. In that cage they have been injected
with hormones and antibiotics, sprayed with disinfectants, and
subjected to artificial cycles of light and darkness. Lodged with

thousands of other birds in a "chicken factory," they have never seen the light of day, let alone an amorous rooster. Many of the cows in the United States do not fare much better. On some dairy farms, milk cows spend much of their lives in barns, chained to stanchions, unable to move, and able only to eat, urinate, defecate, and lactate. On the massive feed lots where many beef cattle are fattened, the animals are immobilized and continuously fed until they are ready for slaughter.

If I buy commercial eggs, chicken, milk, cheese, beef, or other meats, I am tacitly approving and underwriting this treatment of animals. The entrepreneurs who handle animals in this way do so only because there is a demand for the resulting products. Also, if I buy cosmetics and other products which have been tested on animals, I am approving and supporting that cruelty. Thus, though few of us are directly cruel to animals, we condone and support their mistreatment through our market choices.

Moral concern for animals does not require that we become *vegans* (persons who eat no animal foods of any kind) or even vegetarians (persons who abstain from animal flesh). The eating of honey, eggs, cheese, fish, and meat may be necessary to proper human nutrition. In some parts of the world, the use of animal products is necessary to human survival. In northern Scandinavia, for example, only the reindeer kept by the Lapps can turn the tundra grasses into human food—milk and meat.

But moral concern does require that if we use animal products we get them from concerns which treat their animals humanely. There are farms which raise "barnyard chickens." There are dairies whose cows are allowed to roam in the fields and are not treated as biological machines. Moral concern also requires that we avoid cosmetics made by companies which test on animals. It insists that we forego any products whose production involves cruelty to animals. If I am uneasy about animals being trapped in the wilderness for their pelts, then I should not buy a fur coat. The exploitation and destruction of animals would stop in a month if there were no demand for the resulting products.

Most of us use things which cost some creature pain and life. We wear shoes made of cow leather; we enjoy a bowl of fish chowder; we keep warm wearing a sheepskin coat. Even if we cannot or will not forego these products, we should at least feel and express gratitude to the creatures which have suffered on our behalf.

Several years ago I was traveling in provincial Japan and stopped with some business associates at a Japanese inn. For dinner we were served *koi-sashimi* or "raw carp." The whole carp, a reddish brown fish about eighteen-inches long, was presented on a boat-shaped platter. The body was gracefully arched, the head resting on a pillow of white *daikon* radish. Had not slabs of its flesh been arrayed on the plate amidst pieces of raw carrot and radish, I would have sworn the fish had leaped directly from the water to the serving platter. Suddenly, over the top of my sake cup, I saw that the carp's mouth was open and that its chest was expanding and contracting. Aghast, I questioned by companions. They explained that the dish was an example of *ikizukuri*, or "live-carving." The fish has been gutted and filleted but its spinal cord had not been cut. The gasping mouth attested to the freshness of the meat. "Fresh indeed!" I thought, barely able to contain a rising nausea. I have not eaten *ikizukuri* since that time, but each time I eat fish, I try to remember with gratitude the sacrifice made by the creature on my behalf.

Also, our companions on this planet are the billions and billions of plants which form the vegetable kingdom. Algae, mosses, grasses, bushes, and trees germinate, grow, reproduce, and die in almost every corner of the earth.

Plants are necessary to our life, supplying us with both oxygen and food. They have the marvelous ability to take minerals and water from the soil, and carbon dioxide from the air, and with the energy of sunlight, to synthesize the organic compounds— the proteins, carbohydrates, and fats—which we need to sustain life. In doing this they release as a waste product the oxygen we need for our own physical functioning. Until recently plants have been our major, almost sole source of fuel for heating and cooking, of building materials, and of materials for clothing. The vegetable kingdom is a vast and verdant Mother, giving us birth, and feeding, nurturing, and protecting us. Gratitude alone should motivate us to treat plants with respect and even affection.

Plants appear to be inert processors of elements. There is, however, laboratory evidence (much of which appeared first in Dr. Peter Tompkin's *The Secret Life of Plants* published in 1973 by Harper & Row) which indicates that plants are actually highly sensitive energy systems, responding to various stimuli, including music, the human voice, and even human emotion. For example, plants which are lovingly spoken to, and to whom harmonious classical music is played, flourish. The same type of plant in the same physical environment, but subjected to verbal abuse and played rock-and-roll music, sickens and dies. Plants seem able to feel pain, to experience "sympathy" and to anticipate events. When a leaf is cut, there is a change in the electrical field of the plant. If two plants are in a room and one is injured, both will react to this change. And a plant which previously has been cut, will, when a person with a pair of scissors approaches it, exhibit this same pain response.

From the Macrobiotic perspective, however, this understanding of plants is entirely plausible. Plants are living organisms possessing Ch'i or primal energy, operating in highly organized patterns. It is reasonable to think that they have sensitivity and perhaps even a rudimentary consciousness. It is no doubt much different from our own or that of the higher animals, but it warrants our respect and consideration nevertheless. We must treat plants according to the principles of ahimsa and of love.

We should therefore avoid gratuitously injuring or killing a plant. I had a student on an Outward Bound course who had the habit, as we hiked along, of breaking off the tips of tree branches. After a day of watching this, hoping that he would stop on his own, I took him aside. "Glen," I said, "if you were standing quietly next to the trail, minding your own business, and some tree came strolling idly by, and tore off your finger just to have something to hold in its hand, how would you feel?" Glen, albeit a bit thoughtless, was very bright and quickly got the point. Trees along the trail ahead were spared their fingers.

Of course to keep our civilized environment from becoming overgrown, to grow and harvest our food, even to keep our garden and house plants thriving, we must constantly injure and destroy plants. We cut the grass, weed the garden, prune an apple tree, and thin out an exploding azalea. The advocates of "natural agriculture" might disagree, but for most people these are necessary measures and thus not gratuitous and immoral acts. It may be possible, however, to carry out such measures so that the plants "suffer" minimally.

According to some students of vegetable life, plants have the ability, if forewarned that something is about to happen to them, to withdraw their sensitivity. Thus, if we must pick a plant or trim a tree, we can inform it of our intentions. And it may thus be less afflicted by the event. In many traditional cultures, woodsmen, when they were about to cut down a tree, prayed to the spirit of the tree. They announced their intention, apologized for the act, and thanked the tree for its sacrifice. This practice, based on a perception of the consciousness and sacredness of the plant kingdom, is as relevant today as it was centuries ago.

Also, we should treat all plant products with gratitude, care, and respect. In expressing the Law of Reciprocity toward plants, we should never waste anything for which a plant has been destroyed. Every year millions of acres of forest are destroyed to satisfy our appetite for wood and paper products. Paper is so inexpensive and ubiquitous today that we forget that it is produced through the destruction of a living thing (and with considerable pollution of the environment). George Ohsawa was proud that he never wasted even a scrap of paper. He kept used sheets, writing on their clean side. He unglued envelopes and used their hidden spaces for note paper. From this perspective, even buying a massive newspaper like the Sunday *New York Times* can be a moral issue. Most people read only a fraction of the whole thing, but buy and soon discard four or five pounds of newsprint to do so. Literally, huge tracts of land are decimated weekly to keep us in Sunday papers and advertising circulars.

Gratitude and a concern about waste applies especially to

food. Food is the gift of life itself. It represents the sacrifice of the entire vegetable kingdom on behalf of humanity. A moment of silent or spoken gratitude before we eat is a fitting, even a minimal gesture. The Japanese word *Itadakimasu*, uttered before a snack or a meal, means "I humbly receive (this gift of life from nature)." Virtually every culture has a similar prayer or gesture to express gratitude for the food which maintains our life.

Mr. Ohsawa said that to throw away food is a very great sin. It shows that although a plant or animal has given its life for us, we have no awareness or appreciation of that sacrifice. Thus morality requires that we do not waste food. We should save leftovers, and assuming they have not gone bad, eat them later or feed them to a pet. Spoiled food we can add to the garden compost. To waste even a single grain of rice is a violation against the world of nature. As the phrase "One grain, ten thousand grains" suggests, from one grain of rice can come an almost boundless abundance. Thus to waste a single grain is to deprive the future of much bounty.

Existing under, around, and above the plant and animal kingdoms, and making them possible, is the non-organic natural world. This includes the earth itself, with its rocks and soil, the streams, rivers, lakes, seas, and oceans upon it, and the atmosphere of gases enveloping it. It includes too the sun, moon, and other celestial bodies.

Primitive and traditional peoples have viewed this part of the natural world as sacred, and even as possessing feeling and consciousness. Throughout human history, nature as a whole, and particular phenomena within it (certain mountains, rock formations, waterfalls), have been revered and worshipped as divine and conscious realities. The Buddhists of central Asia, for example, consider the earth itself to be alive and conscious. Not wishing to injure it, they do not mine for minerals. And the Japanese mark nearly every mountaintop, waterfall, and place of great natural beauty with a small shrine to honor the indwelling *kami*, or spirit. For the ancient Greeks, the earth was a living, sentient Mother Goddess, known as Gaea.

From the Macrobiotic point of view, nature is indeed sacred and probably has sensibility. Thus the non-organic world, like humans, animals, and plants, must be treated according to the laws of non-injury and of love, implied in the Principle of Reciprocity. Our treatment of the environment is a matter of morality.

By respecting the natural environment and living in harmony with it, human beings can protect and even enhance it. In the Buddhist Himalayas for example, the area surrounding the Zanskar Valley is magnificent but barren. It consists of massive rock faces, overlooking narrow, stony valleys and shallow rivers. Except for an occasional pile of carved Buddhist prayer stones (*mani stones*), there is no sign of humanity. As one comes into the inhabited valley, the low, flat houses of white brick, the stone walls surrounding fields of ripe barley, the white stupas, and the meandering paths add to the beauty of the natural scene. Here, as in fountains and gardens of Versailles, and in the stone garden of Ryoanji temple in Kyoto, we human beings have demonstrated our ability to preserve and enhance the beauties of nature. And in the establishment of wilderness areas and wildlife preserves, we have shown that we can consciously preserve nature even when it goes against immediate economic interest.

We also, alas, have the ability to deface nature, to mar its beauty. We litter parks with plastic bottles and tin cans, we turn meadows into graveyards for rusting automobiles, we block out scenic vistas with billboards, we build tracts of sterile boxlike houses, and we build power lines through pristine wilderness areas.

We have too the ability to brutalize nature, to radically change its structure. And when it suits our purposes we do so. We strip-mine thousands of acres of forest land, cutting trees and peeling away the earth to get at the coal beneath. And we build massive dams, which inundate entire valleys. We also poison the environment. We spray agricultural chemicals on crops, releasing poisons which enter the soil and the water system. We pour factory wastes into rivers and other bodies of water. We release clouds of poisonous gases into the atmosphere. These alien substances so alter the earth's atmosphere, water, and soil, that the plant and animal life dependent on them are threatened.

Human defacement and destruction of the natural environment is not limited to the modern era or to industrialized societies. The ancient Greeks cut down their forests and overgrazed their land with goats. Ground vegetation vanished, rainfall declined, and the peninsula became arid and relatively infertile. A similar process is going on in much of Africa today. But the impact of man on nature in advanced societies is particularly severe. Our massive projects, public and private, change entire landscapes. Chemical pollution undermines the very structure of the natural world. And pollution by radioactive substances does the same but without being perceptible to the senses. The radioactive fallout from the Chernobyl power plant could be neither seen, heard, smelled, nor tasted. Yet it poisoned an immense environmental system. It required that lands be evacuated, that fields be abandoned, and that huge quantities of food be destroyed. And it will affect human, animal, and plant life in northern and central Europe for decades.

It is tempting to think of environmental pollution as something perpetrated by those vast impersonal institutions which control our society. It is the government which builds the radar towers on the tops of mountains, and the dams and the highways. It is agribusiness which saturates farm areas with agricultural poisons and depletes the soil by overuse. It is the paper companies which allow their mills to pour noxious smoke into the air and brown effluent into the streams and rivers. It is the power companies who generate nuclear waste and expose us to the dangers of nuclear accident. It is the oil companies whose ships leak petroleum and devastate the ocean and coastal environments.

These statements are true of course, but they ignore the role that each of us individually plays. We demand and buy the products which necessitate these activities. Every day we use electricity, paper, gasoline, and plastic, and we eat commercially produced food. Also, we elect the officials who approve the dams and are supposed to regulate private industries. We are all deeply, if indirectly, involved in these acts of environmental defacement and destruction.

But we are all also directly involved. Every time I start the engine of my automobile and drive somewhere, use a weed killer on my garden, do the laundry with non-biodegradable soap, pour off some used motor oil onto the ground, I am personally and directly introducing poisons into the environment. Thus every day and probably many times every day, each of us personally contributes to the destruction of the environment.

This violation of the earth, its soil, waters, and sky is so much a part of our daily life that we are scarcely aware of it. To avoid it entirely we would have to radically change our style of living. It is certainly possible. For millennia our ancestors lived very well without electricity, automobiles, and most of the other things which involve us in environmental destruction. And today, in much of the Third World, millions of people are still surviving quite well without the accoutrements of modern industrial life. Yet few of us, Macrobiotic or not, are able or willing to return to an eighteenth century way of life.

Nevertheless, we can bring our relation with the environment more into harmony with the moral Principle of Reciprocity. We can minimize our use of products whose production and/or use involves injury to the non-organic world. And we can use natural, nondestructive alternatives in their stead. For example:

- We can minimize car use. We can walk, bicycle, carpool, or use public transportation whenever possible.
- We can save electricity. We can use air conditioning and electric heat conservatively. We can make sure that lights are not left on in an empty room. We can use mechanical alternatives to electrical devices that consume much energy. For example, the electric lawn mower (like the gas-powered mower) can easily be replaced by a human-powered device. These still are manufactured and work very well. They met people's needs quite adequately for a long time.
- We can garden and farm using organic rather than chemical

methods. There are many successful approaches to organic agriculture. Our ancestors got along without pesticides, herbicides, and artificial fertilizer.

- We can buy food which has been raised organically. There are farmers all over the country who eschew the dead-end practices of chemical agriculture. They produce grains, beans, vegetables, fruits, eggs, milk, cheese, and meat with natural means that sustain rather than destroy the environment. We can support their efforts by seeking out and buying their products, even though they may be more expensive.

- We can use products from natural—hence renewable and relatively non-polluting—materials rather than from synthetics. In Germany there is a *Jute Anstatt Plastik* movement, which promotes the use of burlap, instead of plastic for handbags, shopping bags, and food bags. We can choose a toy made from wood rather than plastic; a sweater made from wool rather than orlon; and a paper bag rather than a plastic one to weigh our produce at the store. If we have a party we can use real plates and cups rather than plastic throwaways.

- We can, whatever the products, use them with respect and care, and without waste. We can reuse paper and plastic bags. We can recycle cans, bottles, and newsprint. We can repair rather than replace appliances and give away outgrown toys and clothing. Every item that continues in use, either in our home or somewhere else, means that there need be one less produced and discarded.

- We can support and be involved in environmental groups, such as the Sierra Club, the Audubon Society, and the World Wildlife Fund, which work to protect the natural environment. Much of the progress made in recent years has been due to such groups.

- We can work for and vote for political candidates and parties who support environmental issues. We "vote" in the supermarket when we buy or do not buy a certain product.

We also vote when we vote—our political choices directly

influence public policy. While the decisions and actions of each of us in our daily life affects the natural environment, those of the government affect it on a massive scale.

Thus our moral lives involve decisions made and actions taken regarding the environment, plants, animals, as well as other human beings. Nearly everything we think, say, and do has a moral or immoral quality. To be a good or moral person requires that we be constantly aware of our thoughts, words, and deeds, and of their implications, immediate and distant. In my treatment of my employees, in my food purchases, even, alas, in my choice of underarm deodorant, I must try to manifest the Principle of Reciprocity.

A question arises of course: Why go through all this trouble? Why commit oneself to constant self-scrutiny, and frequent self-sacrifice? Most of these issues are not covered by the law or by social sanctions. We are unlikely to be indicted for grumbling to the bus driver, or for driving two blocks to the post office. Nor are we likely to be canonized for withholding support from an inhumane dairy industry or for saving and reusing our paper shopping bags.

The reason is threefold. For one thing our good thoughts, words, and deeds help create a happy and harmonious world. That is valuable in itself. But it is also valuable to us since we are part of the world and share in it. If my colleagues at work are happy, in part because I treat them well, I also benefit. If the natural environment is clean, I benefit from it. We think that pollution injures something "out there," but actually it injures us as much as nature. We are only a transformation of the natural environment and every action of pollution is a suicidal one. And if we help keep the air and water clean, we will breath good air and drink good water.

But there are more direct and personal considerations. One is that we are immediately and profoundly affected by the quality of what we think, say, and do. The energy I create and express travels away from me towards its object. But as it goes, it affects my moral body, and every other body—physical, emotional, mental, and spiritual. If my thought, word, or action is a moral one, if it abides by the laws of non-injury and of love, my whole being receives that harmonious, life-giving quality. If I am being immoral, am violating the law of reciprocity, then I am likewise immediately and totally negatively affected. Thus, if I stop on the road to help a disabled motorist I feel, despite the inconvenience involved, a sense of satisfaction and well-being. And when I tell a lie, cheat, or exploit someone, I feel immediately discomfited. In effect, each act is a reward or punishment in itself. And patterns of behavior, moral or immoral, have a long-lasting effect, positive or negative, on every dimension of our lives.

A third consideration is that whatever energy we send into the world ultimately comes back to us. When, for example, I angrily abuse another person, the energy of my words afflicts him, but it does not disperse nor vanish thereafter. It persists as an energy form with my initials on it. Since energy moves spiralically, going away from its point of origin and then back toward it, this energy is a boomerang. Eventually it will return to its source. Hence, whatever we think, say, or do in regard to another—be it a human being, animal, plant, or bit of the environment—comes back to us.

This return "of bread cast upon the waters" can be immediate. Thus the positive energy of a cheery "Good morning" may come back forthwith in the reply, "And a good morning to you, sir." Or it may take a year, or a lifetime. If I choose to drink my coffee from a styrofoam cup every morning and thus take in a little dissolved petrochemical with it, I may not get sick from it for twenty years.

Sometimes the energy of our deeds comes back in a similar, sometimes in an unrecognizable, form. But it always comes back. That is an unavoidable law of the universe. Jesus said, "So whatever you wish that men would do to you, do so to them." (Matthew 7: 12) He might have continued, "because what you do to others will be done to you, and what you do to others you are doing to yourself."

Thus the effort to live a moral, loving life is practical, even prudent. Our thoughts, words, and deeds largely determine what we are and what happens to us. If they are moral and loving, our moral body will be pure and positive, and every other aspect of our being will reflect this. And the world will tend to treat us with that same love and concern. If our thoughts, words, and deeds are selfish and destructive, our moral body and our whole organism will reflect that negative energy. And the world will treat us with that same negativity.

Thus, for our health and happiness, it is important that we cultivate the moral dimension of life. This is not easy. Sloth, inconsideration, insensitivity, and selfishness are all part of human nature. Still there are ways we can make ourselves better persons.

We can develop each of our other bodies. The person who is healthy—physically, emotionally, intellectually, and spiritually— is more likely to be moral and loving. Mr. Ohsawa maintained that a healthy human being is naturally and spontaneously a compassionate and good human being.

We can also cultivate our moral body on the moral and social level itself. We can, for example, associate with people whose moral concern matches our own. And we can avoid people whose patterns of thought, speech, and behavior we do not wish to emulate. "Birds of a feather" do "flock together," but the flock can influence us to change our feathers to conform to it.

Also, we can study and keep before us the teachings and example of the great moral and religious teachers of history and of our own times. The prophet Isaiah, Jesus, the Buddha, Muhammad, Shankara, Albert Schweitzer, Mother Theresa, and many other figures exemplify the moral potential of humankind. By examining carefully their moral teachings and their lives, and by meditating upon these, we can draw energy and inspiration from them.

But the development of the moral life requires more than anything else, self-awareness and self-examination. We must constantly look at our thoughts, words, and actions. We must constantly judge their effect on other people, and on animals, plants, and the world of nature. We must try to cause no harm nor injury. We must strive rather to nurture, support, and love all phenomena. This continuous "moral meditation" is necessary to our health and happiness and thus is an essential part of the Macrobiotic way of life.

7. Twinkle, Twinkle Little Star

There are more things in heaven and earth, Horatio,
Than are dreamt of in your philosophy.
William Shakespeare (1564–1616)

Most of us go through each day engrossed in the affairs of the moment. We get out of bed, eat breakfast, go to work, come home, have dinner, watch TV, read a book, go to bed and fall asleep without giving much thought to greater issues. And we go through our lives in much the same way. We grow up, go to school, get a job, get married, have children, retire, and eventually die. There is usually something to do, to be entertained by, or to worry about. We seldom have the time or the inclination to consider the basic circumstances of our existence. We seldom trouble about the fact that we live in a universe which (to borrow Churchill's description of the Soviet Union) is "a riddle wrapped in a mystery inside an enigma."

At some point, though, we each awaken to the bare reality of our situation, our "human condition." We see that we are small, mortal creatures on a spinning orb in a vast and incomprehensible universe. We realize that we do not know how or why the universe came to be, nor how or why we came to exist in it.

This experience may come to us spontaneously, as we walk alone on a windswept beach, or gaze upward at the starry immensity of space. It may come with an emotional shock, the death of a parent perhaps. Whatever the circumstances, we are likely to feel awe-struck and helpless, and then we are likely to try to answer the questions which overwhelm us. We strive to make sense of it all. We ask ourselves "How did the universe come to be? How did I come to exist in it? Does my life have any meaning or purpose? What happens after death?" We struggle for answers, appealing to our religious training, to our common sense, and to our knowledge of philosophy. Probably this struggle will not last long. Our moment of silence or of grief passes and we are drawn back into the distractions and pressures of daily life.

It is important though that we continue this effort to answer the basic questions of life. An *ideology* is a clear and systematic understanding of the universe and of human life and destiny. It is a necessary part of life, especially for a person who aspires to be healthy or whole. Even amidst the distractions and busyness of life, we must wrestle with the elemental questions and formulate an ideology. We must nourish and exercise our "ideological body." As Socrates said, "The unexamined life is not worth living."

Every human culture has struggled with the basic issues of existence, and has expressed the resulting ideology in mythology, religious doctrines, and in philosophy. Thus throughout human history the typical individual received a clear and specific ideology as part of his cultural birthright. Born into a Jewish, Christian, Buddhist, or animist family, he was taught the corresponding world view from an early age. Often this belief system was shared by all members of the immediate community and even by the society as a whole. Very likely it was sanctioned by the state and promulgated by an official religious body.

Even today in many parts of the world, the typical person inherits a specific ideology. In the more traditional societies of the Third World, and wherever traditional religion is strong, he is taught a view of the world shared by his family, and perhaps by his community and nation. In the Marxist nations he is presented with an official state ideology. When and if he is struck by the riddle of the human condition, the bequeathed ideology helps both in framing the questions and in answering them.

However, many people today, particularly in the secular societies of the West, have no clear ideological inheritance. They grow up in families with no religious orientation or with a nominal one only. They receive no religious or philosophical instruction in school. They may be exposed to a national ideology but it is rather vague and not actively promoted. Thus even as educated adults, they may never have confronted the basic issues of life, nor have studied even one ideology which tries to answer them. So, when the human condition inevitably confronts them, they are ill-prepared. They have no ideology to which even to refer. They may not know even the questions to ask, let alone the possible answers to them.

To develop health in the ideological body, we must (if we do not have one already) formulate a satisfying ideology. To do this we need first to know the critical questions to be asked. We need also to know the various answers which humanity has given to these questions.

In his book *Unmasking the New Age* (Intervarsity Press, Downer's Grove, Illinois, 1986), Douglas Groothuis lists the questions which a valid ideology must answer. These include:

- How did the universe come to exist? If there is an Absolute Creator, what is its relation to the created universe? Thus an ideology has a *metaphysics*.
- How do we human beings know what we know about the universe? Thus an ideology has an *epistemology*, or "theory of knowledge."
- What is the nature of "human nature?" Is it good, bad, or indifferent? Thus an ideology has an *anthropology*, or "view of human nature."
- What is the source of human problems and suffering? Thus an ideology has a *demonology*.
- What is the way to end human suffering? Thus an ideology has a *soteriology*, or "theory of salvation."
- What is the nature of time and to what goal, if any, is history moving? Thus an ideology has a theory of time and a collective *eschatology*, literally a view of "the last things."
- What is the destiny of the individual human being? Thus an ideology has a personal eschatology, or "a view of the goal of individual life."
- What is going to happen in history? Thus an ideology has a general eschatology, or "a view of the nature of time and of the end to which history is moving."
- What is the value of other and different points of view, especially those propounded by religious leaders and con-

tained in the religions which developed from them? Thus an ideology has an *ecclesiology*, or "a view of religion."

There are three broad ideologies into which the various religions and philosophies fall. These are the *theistic, pantheistic,* and *atheistic.* To each major ideological issue these three give distinct and different answers.

The *theistic* world view is held by the principal Western religions—Judaism, Christianity, and Islam. While these three faiths differ on particular points, they share a basically similar view of God, nature, and of the human being. The Christian version of the theistic world view is espoused by about one-quarter of the world's population.

The metaphysics of the orthodox Christian world view is based on a single, absolute deity or God—eternal, infinite, and all-knowing. This God is personal in that "He" exists, functions, and is conscious in a way similar to that of a human individual or "person." God wills and acts. He experiences emotions of anger and of love, and has plans for humanity and the world.

God has created all that exists—the heavens, earth, plants, animals, and human beings—*ex nihilo* ("out of nothing"). He continues to sustain the universe. Without Him it would cease to be. The power, wisdom, and majesty of God are reflected in His creation. But God is distinct and separate from His creation just as a potter is distinct and separate from the pots he fashions from clay. There is an unfathomable gulf between God and the creation.

God wishes that humanity know about Him and about His will. Therefore He has revealed Himself in history through the Hebrew prophets and then in the person and teachings of Jesus Christ. These revelations of the divine nature and will are contained in the Holy Scriptures.

Human beings, though made in the image of God, have a fallen nature due to the pride and disobedience of Adam and Eve. Hence human beings are by nature proud, selfish, and corrupt. They cannot help but violate the divine commandments.

This willful disobedience to God's law is the cause of all human suffering.

Human salvation lies in accepting the gift of divine grace, with which comes forgiveness and the possibility of moral improvement. In the person of Christ, God has expiated the sins of the first man and woman and of all humanity. Reconciled to God, human beings can begin to live according to God's law of love.

Time is linear, moving straight in one direction. Thus history has begun at a particular point (the Creation) and is moving toward a conclusion. This is the Second Coming of Christ when the world will be transformed and a new and blessed age under Christ's sovereignty will begin.

The history of each individual is also linear. Each person, depending on his response to the offer of grace and the demand for obedience, will be judged after death. Each will spend eternity either in painful separation from God (hell) or in blissful communion with Him (heaven).

The life and sacrifice of Jesus, the "man-God" is a unique event in history. Thus, only the Church founded on Him and His teachings, has the complete truth and the means for human salvation. Other religious leaders and teachings may have part of the truth but only a part. For this reason Christians over the centuries have tried to convert others to their faith.

This orthodox Christian world view of course is just one version of the theistic ideology. Some Christians differ with it on the literal truth of the Bible, on the relation between Jesus and God, and on other issues. Jews and Muslims reject its understanding of Jesus's identity and function. But most Christians, Jews, and Muslims agree on its fundamental beliefs. The broad theistic ideology has been an important world view, particularly in Western and Near Eastern civilization, for over two millennia. Theistic ideas exist in the East, among certain Hindu and Buddhist sects for example, but they are secondary in importance.

The second broad ideology is the *pantheistic*. This understanding of the universe is the basis for most of the religions of the Orient. Hinduism, Taoism, Shinto, and to some degree Buddhism, are all pantheistic. It has existed also in the West as a "minority voice." Pantheism has been present in the thought of Pythagoras; Epictetus; the Essenes (a Hebrew ascetic group active during the time of Christ); the Jewish Kabbala; Meister Eckhart (a twelfth century German monk and mystic); the European Romantics, including Wordsworth, Goethe, and Heine; the American Transcendentalists, including Emerson and Thoreau; and of the Theosophical Movement, which in the last century introduced Eastern religious ideas and practices into the West.

The basis of pantheistic metaphysics is a Universal Spirit, infinite and eternal, which encompasses all that exists. This Universal Spirit is non-personal, lacking particular intent, feeling, and thought.

The phenomenal universe is created as a spontaneous out-pouring of this Universal Spirit. All creation, in its material and nonmaterial forms, is a transformation of the Absolute. Every object and creature therefore is a manifestation of God. God equals the universe. The universe equals God.

The human being is the most developed manifestation of the Universal Spirit. In the human being the finite universe becomes self-aware, and recognizes its identity with God. Each person then is in essence "a sleeping God," a spiritual being with infinite potential for understanding and accomplishment.

The reason we human beings, in spite of our divine nature, suffer, is that we do not remember who we are, and we do not tap our true potential. We need only to look within and we will discover the spark of divinity and the source of all truth. Various spiritual practices, such as meditation and yoga, can help us release our inner, hidden divinity.

For the pantheist, time and history are cyclical. They move in cycles but perhaps with a generally upward evolutionary trend. The universe as a whole and all phenomena within it emerge from the Universal Spirit, go through cycles of change and transformation, and ultimately return to their source.

The individual soul also follows a cyclical path. It emerges from the universal ocean of being like a single drop of watery spray, and goes through various incarnations—manifestations in human and other forms. In each incarnation it learns something essential to its evolution. Thus the death of the individual is an illusion, only the putting off of one fleshly garment before the putting on of another. When the individual soul has at last fully remembered its divine nature, it returns to the perfect bliss, knowledge, and being of the Godhead. Eventually it may repeat the cycle of emergence, evolution, and return. This is the "play" or amusement of the Universal Spirit.

Pantheism tends to view all religions as true and valuable. The universal truths can be expressed in a variety of ways, all of them valid. It is as if the various religious founders had been standing in different places at the base of a great mountain. From the summit shone a magnificent light, the light of the Universal Spirit. Each was attracted to that light and began to climb the mountain. Depending on his particular vantage point, that leader's description and name for the summit varied. Hence theistic, pantheistic, and even polytheistic religions developed, each with its own name for the Universal Spirit—Yahweh, God, Allah, Brahman, the Tao, the Cosmic Buddha. Also, depending on that leader's route up the mountain, his understanding of the path to the summit varied. Thus, some religions emphasize obedience to the law, some the receiving of grace through sacraments, some prayer, and others physical austerities or meditation. All religious practices are valid in that they make possible humanity's ascent to the divine. Thus, all religions spring from a common experience and aspiration, and each deserves credence and respect. A religion may be especially well-suited to a certain person or culture, but each is valid in its own way.

Over the last twenty years pantheistic ideas have become more familiar and widespread in the West. Various Oriental religions and religious practices—Yoga, Transcendental Meditation, Hare Krishna, Tai Chi Ch'uan, Aikido, Karate, Judo, Sufism—have been embraced by substantial numbers of people. Also, Western pantheism, as contained in the Kabbala, astrology, and other aspects of the New Age ideology, has had a revival.

The third broad ideology is the *atheistic*. Ideologies which deny the existence of an Absolute Spirit and of a spiritual element in man existed in ancient Greece. But since the development of empirical science in the sixteenth century and the rationalistic Enlightenment of the seventeenth century, the atheistic-materialistic ideology has had a strong influence in the West and around the world. It asserts that only what can be perceived through the senses, and which has mass and dimension, is real.

From this materialistic perspective then, God, who cannot be seen, heard, felt, or measured, does not exist. He is a superstition created by humanity as it seeks comfort and meaning in a difficult and meaningless world. The universe is self-existent, consisting of matter and energy manifesting in an infinite number of interacting phenomenon. The concepts of infinity and eternity, being beyond our finite intellect, are irrelevant abstractions.

In this arbitrary universe, various forms of life—plant, animal, and then human—have emerged through the process of evolution. The human being, then, is an evolved animal controlled largely by animal needs and passions and subject to the vagaries of nature. But through evolution the human being has acquired the power of reason. Employing this reason in science, the human being can understand himself and the world around him. Employing it in technology, he can control and change his environment and himself. Thus, in the natural and social sciences and in the technologies derived from them, lies hope for human progress.

The atheistic ideology sees time and history moving in a linear fashion. History is controlled, however, not by a divine hand but by chance and by human will and action. And it is moving not toward a heavenly kingdom but toward an earthly Utopia made possible by science and technology. The life of the individual human being is likewise linear, but there is no life after death. Death terminates the existence of the person.

From the atheistic point of view, the various religions are equally false. They are based on superstitions, on unfounded beliefs in an absolute spiritual being, the immortality of the human soul, salvation, and life after death. Religions may contain moral principles which stabilize individual and social life.

But they contain little else of value. Religions make people passive and distract them from the task of improving life in this world. And they have been used through history by the rich and powerful to pacify and exploit the poor.

The broad atheistic ideology includes a variety of viewpoints. On one end of its spectrum there is, for example, Marxist-Leninism. This "atheistic" communism maintains (against all evidence to the contrary) that human reason and hard work can create a Utopian society. In this worker's paradise there will be no need of a central government; each person will work according to his ability and receive according to his needs. The *nihilist-hedonist* ideology is quite different on certain points. This maintains that since there is no God, no human spirit, and no afterlife, the only value in life is the pleasure we experience from moment to moment. The pursuit of individual pleasure then is the chief aim of human existence.

One of the major world religions is based on an ideology which does not focus on a transcendent reality. Siddhartha Gautama, the founder of Buddhism, taught that the primary concern of the human being should be to escape suffering. He said that the existence of God, of a human spirit, and of life after death, are unfathomable and extraneous issues. Every human being is like a person shot with a poison arrow. His priority should be getting the arrow out, not in finding out who shot it, where it was made, and what kind of poison was smeared on its tip. Thus, as the Buddha ("He who has awakened"), Gautama taught a practical path of ethical behavior and meditational introspection, designed to end suffering. He avoided metaphysical issues. In time, Buddhism became a religion in the usual sense. The Buddha came to be identified with the Absolute Spirit, and doctrines of salvation and life after death appeared. But in its original form, Buddhism was a pragmatic way of life, based on an ideology which did not concern itself with a cosmic deity or Universal Spirit.

The three broad ideologies (theistic, pantheistic, and atheistic), with their many variations, include, then, a wide variety of ways of looking at and understanding the world. These are a rich resource in the task of developing a coherent and satisfying view of life.

Each of us should study this wonderful heritage of human insight and wisdom. If we have no clear ideology, such study will help us develop one. If we are dissatisfied with our view of the world and want to amend or change it, such study will help us in that task. Even if we have a developed and satisfying ideology it will serve us well. What is said of languages is true also of ideologies—that to know only one is to know none.

We should become, in effect, students of religion and philosophy. We should study our own tradition and the religious heritage of other peoples. The systematic study of ideology is not the monopoly of university students, academics, writers, clergy, and other intellectuals. Every person can and should struggle with the basic issues of life, can and should formulate a satisfying and coherent ideology or view of the world.

This endeavor can involve a variety of activities. They include:

- Studying one's own tradition in depth, informally or perhaps formally, in academic or church courses and in retreat programs.
- Reading books, watching programs, taking courses on the religions of the world.
- Discussing with friends, acquaintances, and strangers, particularly those of other faiths, what exactly they believe.
- Periodically carefully considering each of the basic areas of ideology, deciding exactly what one believes regarding each, and even writing that belief down in a clear, coherent manner.

Our ideological body, then, is an important factor in our life. Our health as a complete human being depends on its vigor and full development as much as it depends on the vitality of our physical or emotional body. The person with no clear beliefs about the universe and his place in it is pitiful indeed. He has failed to develop that self-awareness which is perhaps a unique attribute of the human being. We must then take time and energy to nourish and exercise this aspect of our humanity. We must do this consciously, carefully, and throughout our lives.

For each human being the "ideological task" presents a real challenge. For the Western person interested in or involved in Macrobiotics it presents an especially difficult challenge. This is because Macrobiotics possesses an "official" ideology—a particular East Asian expression of pantheism—which probably is quite different from the world view on which he has been raised.

The Macrobiotic ideology, developed by Mr. Ohsawa and carried on and elaborated by later leaders of the movement (Kushi, Aihara, Tomio Kikuchi of Brazil, et al.), is based on traditional Yin-Yang thinking. It views the important ideological issues as follows:

The universe is the spontaneous manifestation of the Tao, an impersonal universal absolute, and operates according to the laws of alternating opposites.

We human beings are the culmination of evolution. Thus our human nature is basically good and we are destined for health and happiness. Human suffering is caused by our failure to recognize our place in nature and to abide by nature's laws. Our mistakes in the choice and preparation of food are particularly critical. We can end our suffering and realize our birthright of health by living in harmony with the natural order.

The first and necessary step is to follow the principle of ecological eating. We should eat a diet in harmony with the environment—in most situations, one based on locally grown whole grains and seasonal vegetables. We human beings have various dimensions however, sensory, emotional, intellectual, social, ideological, and spiritual. Each is important in itself and each is related to all the others. So we must cultivate each of these bodies. We must bring every part of our life into harmony with the order of the universe. If we do so we can realize boundless health and happiness.

Since the human being is the highest manifestation of the universe and of the Tao, its ultimate destiny is to return to the source of all. Our individual death is not final. When we die we return to the world of pure spirit, perhaps to return to the Tao, perhaps, if necessary, to incarnate again.

Human history is cyclical, without beginning and without end. The world goes through cycles of creation and prosperity (Yang) and of dissolution (Yin). The present period, while one in which the forces of chaos seem to reign, is about to change to one of universal order, peace, and prosperity. Macrobiotics will play a major role in the establishment of this New Age.

Finally, according to the Macrobiotic ideology, all religions are expressions of dialectical monism. Each presents in its own vocabulary the same basic world view as that expressed in the Taoist theory of Yin and Yang. Properly understood, Judaism, Christianity, and Islam, as well as the pantheistic faiths, express the same fundamental truths as does the Macrobiotic ideology. Moses, Jesus, and Muhammad were really teachers of the Unique Principle.

This Macrobiotic world view is a coherent and powerful ideology. And it aspires to being an all-embracing one. But it is nevertheless a particular ideology. It differs with the Jewish and Christian versions of theism on several important points. And it differs also with the atheistic-materialist world view on several major issues. The question arises therefore, is Macrobiotics compatible with Christianity, Judaism, Islam, and atheism. Can one be a Christian Macrobiotic (or Macrobiotic Christian), a Jewish Macrobiotic, or an atheistic Macrobiotic?

It may be argued that to be Macrobiotic one must accept the entire Macrobiotic ideology, including its Taoist views of the universe, human nature, destiny, and salvation; and that therefore a true Macrobiotic cannot be an orthodox Jew or Christian, or an atheistic scientist. I believe though, that one can be fully Christian and Macrobiotic, Jewish and Macrobiotic, and scientific and Macrobiotic.

Certainly there are major points of differences, on metaphysics, epistemology, eschatology, and soteriology. But much of the essence of Macrobiotics—its vision of human health, its respect for food, its holistic approach to health—is not intrinsically related to these ideological issues. The Christian or Jewish world view can support and include most of "the heart of the Macrobiotic artichoke," as well as the pantheistic ideology can.

Back in Chapter 2 we presented the seven concepts essential to Macrobiotics. Stated briefly they are:

1. The universe is an infinitely diverse but monistic and integrated organism constantly in flux according to dialectical and orderly patterns.
2. The human being is a microcosm of the macrocosm and thus also is a diverse, but ultimately monistic and integrated organism.
3. Human health or wholeness is the full and harmonious development of the human organism, including each of its various bodies.
4. Health is the natural birthright of the human being and the realization of this birthright is our own responsibility.
5. Diet is one, very important, factor in achieving health.
6. The optimal diet is an ecologically based one, consisting of foods naturally and abundantly present in the immediate environment.
7. The path to true health must include a proper diet, but must include as well, the conscious and insightful cultivation of each area of life, from physical to spiritual.

From the Jewish point of view, the main difficulty lies in the explanation of point number one. The Absolute is described as a pantheistic and non-personal Infinite Expansion, or Tao. This is simply not the same as Yahweh, the God of the Israelites, who creates the world, rules it, chooses His people, and guides and chastises them through history. Yahweh is personal, distinct from creation, but active in history. Ohsawa's Tao is impersonal, immanent, and "is" history.

But one can put Yahweh in the place of the Tao, and still retain Yin and Yang and the Unique Principle. The laws of Yin and Yang describe how the universe operates; they do not explain how the universe came into being. And even in the creation story in Genesis, Yahweh creates by a process of bifurcation, of division into opposite pairs—Light and Darkness, Heaven and Earth, Man and Woman.

The other statements do not raise serious problems. In fact, they reflect Jewish attitudes on the issues. The ancient Hebrews recognized the profound relationship between body and spirit. The Hebrew word *ru'ach* refers to both "breath" and "spirit." The Israelites believed that human health and happiness are possible if the laws of God are obeyed. Suffering results from disobedience to the divine law, and repentance and the cessation of suffering are always possible.

Diet has always played an important role in Jewish life. A number of laws in the Torah (the first five books of the Jewish Bible) concern dietary practice. The observance of these regulations, designed to maintain a *kosher* ("clean") diet, has been central to Jewish culture.

The ancient Hebrews even understood the central importance of grains. According to Genesis 1, Yahweh says to Adam and Eve, "Behold I have given you every plant yielding seed which is upon the face of all the earth, and every tree with seed in its fruit. And you shall have them for food." Though after the Fall and the Flood, God amends this injunction, the Jews remembered the importance of cereals. During the Babylonian Captivity (sixth century B.C.) Daniel and other Hebrew youths are serving in the king's court. Nebuchadnezzar offers them the rich food of his table but they choose instead a simple diet of pulses (grains and beans). After ten days the Hebrews are obviously stronger and healthier than the native youths who had eaten rich food.

The idea that every aspect of human life must conform to divine law (in Macrobiotic terms, the "order of the universe") is also basic to Jewish life. The Talmud, the writings governing Jewish life, treat every dimension of existence—physical, intellectual, social, moral, legal, and spiritual.

Thus, for an orthodox or conservative Jew, it can be easy to understand and adopt Macrobiotic theory and practice. For a reformed Jew, whose liberal theology may verge on pantheism, it can be even easier. It is not surprising, then, that many Jewish

people have been active in Macrobiotics since its introduction to
the West. Some of these, stimulated by Macrobiotics to re-
evaluate their own tradition, have renounced secularism and
become devout practitioners of their ancient faith.

For the devout Christian the issues are a bit more complex.
Like the Jew, he cannot accept an impersonal, pantheistic Absolute. The personal, loving God of the New Testament, who
incarnates as Jesus Christ, and suffers on the cross for the sins
of humanity, is not the same as Ohsawa's "Infinite Expansion."
But the Christian, like the Jew, can resolve this by substituting
his personal God for the pantheistic Absolute. And he also can
do so while retaining the law of opposites. As the Reverend
John Ineson points out in his book, *The Way of Life: Macrobiotics and the Spirit of Christianity* (Japan Publications, 1986),
the New Testament as well as the Old contains many examples
of the "dualistic-complementary" thinking described in the
Unique Principle. For example, in the Beatitudes of Matthew 4,
the thoughts, "Blessed are the poor in spirit for theirs is the
Kingdom of God. . . . Blessed are the meek for they shall inherit
the earth. . . ." express beautifully the eternal cycle of opposites
which is at the heart of Macrobiotic thinking. The terms Yin
and Yang are foreign to the New Testament and to the Christian
tradition. But one can substitute another more familiar pair of
terms, Expansion and Contraction, or Alpha and Omega, and
not compromise the basic idea.

But for the orthodox Christian there is another problem area
in the heart of the Macrobiotic artichoke. It concerns human
nature, and its ability to abide by the laws of God and nature.

According to the Macrobiotic world view, health and happiness are the natural birthright of the human being. We suffer
because we fail to live in harmony with the order of nature.
Since human nature is basically good, we need only to be
reminded of the Tao. Knowing the way, we will be able to follow it and will realize our human wholeness.

The orthodox Christian can agree that health is the natural
condition of the human being. A loving God created humanity
not to suffer but to rejoice in the creation. And he can agree that

we suffer because we do not obey the laws of God and nature. But the Christian must disagree regarding our ability to rectify our lives. For him, human nature is fallen and corrupt. Even knowing the good, we do not do it. As Jesus said, "The spirit is willing but the flesh is weak." To change our way of living, to live in obedience to the laws of God and nature requires a total transformation of human nature. And that transformation, while it can begin within us, requires help to complete. It requires the transforming grace of God.

For the orthodox Christian the other central Macrobiotic ideas present little difficulty. He can agree that the human being is an integrated organism, and that proper diet affects its well-being. He can readily accept also the principle of ecological eating. That God has put the most appropriate foods for us in our immediate environment is an expression of divine love. He can also understand the importance of grains. Did not Jesus choose bread as a symbol for his own divine body? And he can agree that health requires a careful nurturing of each dimension of life. But the Christian cannot accept the idea that unassisted, we can follow the path to health and happiness. He must affirm that in order to obey the laws of nature and God we need God's forgiveness, love, and transforming grace.

This is a serious, but not fatal obstacle to the Christian's adoption of Macrobiotics. It requires though, that item four in the Macrobiotic "heart" be amended to include the concept of divine grace. Instead of asserting our absolute responsibility for our lives and health, it might affirm that "We human beings create ourselves, our health, and our lives by what we think, say, and do. We can change ourselves so that our lives issue in health and happiness but it requires in addition to our own effort, the grace and help of God."

For the liberal Christian, for the Unitarian or Quaker, for example, the embracing of Macrobiotic thought and practice may not require even these changes. His theology may be close to pantheism. His view of human nature, less affected by the idea of original sin, may be more positive. And he may rely on human effort rather than grace and the hand of God for the transformation of human life.

It is possible, then, to be both Christian and Macrobiotic. The ideological adjustments necessary for the orthodox believer are substantial, but they leave the heart of Macrobiotic thought and practice intact. And they add concepts, that of a personal God and of transforming grace, which may indeed be an enrichment rather than a compromise of the Macrobiotic world view.

For an atheist, a rigorous scientist for example, the full Macrobiotic ideology poses many problems. Its pantheistic metaphysics, its largely deductive approach to knowledge, its spiritual view of human nature and destiny, all clash with an empirical approach to reality. But the essential elements of the Macrobiotic "artichoke heart" involve few difficulties. Most of these ideas were, until recently, alien and even absurd to the strict, materialistic scientist. Today however, largely corroborated by scientific research, they are increasingly familiar to the scientist and are likely to be part of his own world view.

For example, Ohsawa's Unique Principle describes a monistic universe in which all opposites, such as matter and energy, and time and space, are simply forms of one another. Matter is compacted energy; energy is diffuse and rapidly moving matter. Since the formulation of Einstein's Theory of Relativity and the development of quantum physics, it is increasingly obvious to scientists that matter and energy are indeed forms of one another.

Similarly, scientific research has been discovering the integrated nature of the human being. Though long tied to a dualistic understanding of the body and mind, science is recognizing that the two are interrelated and interdependent. The new field of psycho-neuro-immunology, for example, is based on the realization that emotions, thoughts, and mental attitudes deeply affect both resistance to disease and the ability to recover from illness.

Meanwhile, medical and nutritional research are corroborating Macrobiotic ideas about diet and health. The current consensus in the medical community is that at least thirty-five percent of all cancers are caused by poor diet. The dietary recommendations of the American Heart Association and the American Cancer Society now warn against refined carbohydrates (sugar and white flour) and excess animal protein and fats (fatty red meats, eggs, and dairy foods). They promote whole grains, fish, and fresh vegetables and fruits. Every year these recommendations sound more and more like the Standard Macrobiotic Diet!

From the Macrobiotic point of view this is not at all surprising. Macrobiotics has tended to stress an intuitive and a deductive (from general principles to specifics) approach to knowledge. In part, this was a reaction against the strict scientism of Western culture. But Macrobiotics accepts the validity of the inductive or scientific approach. If the ideas and practices of Macrobiotics are indeed true, then scientific studies and the accumulation of data will validate them.

In any case, the central tenets of Macrobiotics are increasingly acceptable to the scientific mind. And indeed many physicians and scientists are studying and practicing Macrobiotics today.

Even the most conservative and skeptical scientist, without compromising his world view, can embrace and practice Macrobiotics. He can do so by approaching Macrobiotics as a set of hypotheses about human health, hypotheses which need to be tested. Thus he may say:

"I will assume that the laws of Yin and Yang are valid, that the human organism is totally integrated, and that health—the full development of each aspect of that organism—is a viable possibility. I will also assume that food is an important factor in the realization of health and that an ecological diet based on whole grains and vegetables is optimal for human health. And I will assume that the cultivation of each dimension of life is important. And making all these assumptions, I will act according to them. I will eat a broad Macrobiotic diet, wear cotton undershorts, learn to play the ukulele, study Ukrainian architecture, be kind to plants, and do all the other things an upstanding, well-rounded Macrobiotic person is supposed to do.

After a year, my level of health and happiness will verify these assumptions or it will not."

For the scientist then, and for others holding an atheistic (or agnostic) viewpoint, ideology is not an obstacle to the practice of Macrobiotics. The Marxist-Leninist, the nihilist, the ethical humanist, each can embrace and practice Macrobiotics as something largely verified by scientific research, or as a possibly valid "working hypothesis." For the Marxist especially, the Macrobiotic world view should be very interesting. The Unique Principle with its dialectic of Yin and Yang is very similar to the Hegelian dialectical philosophy on which Marxism is based.

Those people with a broad pantheistic world view will have little difficulty with the Macrobiotic ideology. The world view underlying Hinduism, Mahayana Buddhism, Taoism, Confucianism, and the nature-oriented religions of "nonliterate" peoples (Aborigines, Bushmen, Navajo), is very similar to that of Macrobiotics. For followers of these faiths, even the full Macrobiotic ideology is quite familiar and acceptable. And many or all of the elements of the "artichoke heart" likewise are familiar and acceptable. Thus in the West, many practitioners of Indian religious disciplines, such as Yoga and meditation, of the martial arts, such as Aikido, T'ai ch'i Chuan, and Karate, and of Zen meditation, practice Macrobiotics as well. And where Macrobiotics exists in a culture dominated by a pantheistic world view (i.e. that of Japan), there has been no conflict.

According to some teachers of Macrobiotics, ideology is a product of food. A diet of whole grains (eaten in their unbroken form), supplemented by beans and vegetables, leads to holistic, that is, pantheistic thinking. A diet of broken and ground grains (bread and other flour products), supplemented by animal foods, leads to dualistic or theistic thinking. Thus, Western theism, with its emphasis on a personal God, on original sin, on grace, on heaven and hell, is the result of centuries of bread-and-meat eating. According to this view, as we eat a diet of whole, unbroken grains, and of beans and vegetables, our thinking naturally will become less theistic and more pantheistic.

This may indeed happen. It may however not happen. In the

West, our ancestors for centuries have held theistic beliefs. We may find that though we eat boiled grains rather than bread, and tofu and tempeh rather than meat, eggs, and cheese, we will continue to hold these beliefs. A personal and loving God, our own moral weakness, and the need for forgiveness and grace may continue to be real for us. Just as certain foods are appropriate to certain environments and their people, certain ideas and ideologies may also be best suited for certain areas and peoples. And if we do doggedly persist in being Christian, Jewish, Muslim, or atheist, we will not be any less Macrobiotic for it.

Thus, Macrobiotics contains a very specific ideology. This has a metaphysics, expressed in particular concepts and terms, and also a distinct view of human nature, of human suffering and salvation, of history and of human destiny. One can accept and adopt this ideology in its entirety. But this is not necessary in order to practice and to benefit from Macrobiotics. One can embrace the basic principles of Macrobiotics and apply them in one's daily life, without becoming a Taoist and pantheist. One can remain (or later become) a Jew, a Christian, Muslim, agnostic, atheist, Buddhist, Hindu, or anything else one chooses to be.

In the Macrobiotic way of life, dealing seriously with the issue of ideology is much more important than accepting a particular world view. We can become happy and healthy without adopting the Macrobiotic ideology. But we cannot become happy and healthy unless we take seriously the underlying questions of existence.

Thus we must consider each ideological issue. We must study the various ways each can be resolved. We must consult our own experience and intuition. We must formulate clear, coherent, and satisfying opinions of our own. And we must do this periodically throughout our lives. Only in this way can we realize that wholeness in our ideological body essential to our development as healthy and happy human beings.

8. Into the Arms of the Infinite

Wherein lies happiness? In that which becks
Our ready minds to fellowship divine,
A fellowship with essence; till we shine
Full alchemized and free of space. Behold
The clear religion of heaven!
John Keats (1795–1821)

We human beings share a common situation. Viewed objectively, it is a difficult and even painful one. This human condition is basically one of limitation.

We are limited, for example, in terms of time. We begin to exist independently at a point in time—the moment of our birth. Thereafter we grow, mature, reach the peak of our physical and mental powers, then decline, die, and disappear. By all indications, we are a temporary phenomena, "a vanity of vanities."

We are limited also in terms of space. While the earth on which we live is relatively vast and the heavens extend around it apparently without end, physically we are but a tiny speck of matter. We move, but rather slowly. We can be only in one place at a time. We cannot occupy the same space as another person or object.

We are limited as well in terms of pleasure. We have many needs and desires—for food, sex, power, wealth, and fame. We feel pleasure when we satisfy them. But our satisfaction is only temporary. Our hungers always return, insistent on being satisfied. Often we cannot fulfill our desires and we feel the pain of frustration. Often we do fulfill them, but then we lose that which satisfies our desire and we feel the pain of loss. Our lives, then, are a ceaseless alternation of pleasure and pain, satisfaction and frustration, gain and loss. The joy and laughter in the world seem roughly in balance with the sorrow and weeping.

Also, we are limited in terms of knowledge and understanding. Our intellect can comprehend many of the phenomena in the world. But before the mystery of the universe and of existence itself, it must stand humble and dumb. The intellect is a finite instrument which cannot grasp the infinite size and complexity of the universe. However well-educated and insightful we may be, if on a clear, starry night, we gaze up at the sky and try to comprehend that the heavens continue endlessly in all directions, we simply cannot do it. And if we try to comprehend that there are billions of cells in our own body, that within each there are billions of molecules, and that at every moment in these cells and involving these molecules, there are countless chemical reactions occurring which make life possible, again our intellect must acknowledge its impotence.

We then are tiny, sluggish, somewhat befuddled creatures rooted on our spinning home in what may be a very second-rate neighborhood in the universe. Confronting this situation, we try to figure it out. Using our experience, reason, intuition, and the insights and revelations of the past, we try to formulate a satisfactory world view.

From this attempt to comprehend come three broad ideologies. One of these, the atheistic-materialistic, bravely affirms that what seems to be true is indeed true. Yes, it says, the world, we, and our lives are what they appear to be. The universe is a random, conglomerate of matter and energy. We are animals who have evolved a mental faculty. Like other animals, we are born, we suffer, and we die. Life is, as it most plainly seems to be, "nasty, brutish, and short." The best we can do is, by using our intellect, to make it as comfortable as possible. The French Existentialist philosophers of the post-World War II period took this view as the starting point of their thought. They maintained that given *la condition humaine*, the first issue any aware human being must confront is that of suicide.

The two other broad ideologies, the theistic and the pantheistic, however, maintain that there is more here than meets the eye. The theistic world view affirms the existence of a transcendent, personal Being, who is the creator of the universe, and who is infinite, eternal, all-knowing, and full of light and joy. It affirms too the existence of a human spirit or soul, created by the Creator and possessing potential for everlasting life. And it maintains that the end of human life is not death. Rather, human destiny lies in the communion after death of the soul with the divine being. In this blissful apprehension of God, the *visio Dei*, or "vision of God" (described by Dante in the last chapter of *The Divine Comedy*), the human soul shares in the eternal and infinite joy of the divine being.

Pantheism likewise posits a transcendent reality, also eternal, infinite, radiant, and perfectly blissful. In the Hindu tradition for example, Brahman is described as *sat* ("pure being"), *chit* ("pure knowledge"), and *ananda* ("pure joy"). Pantheism sees the individual human soul as identical with and part of this Universal Spirit. *Atman* (the individual soul) equals Brahman and each human being moves toward blissful and eternal union with the Infinite.

Theism and pantheism, then, although they differ on particulars, share several crucial ideas: there is a transcendent reality; the human being has an eternal soul; human destiny involves a union or communion of the soul with the transcendant. Both may be called therefore "religious" ideologies.

The term "religious" and its parent noun "religion" are often misunderstood. They have a variety of negative connotations. Many people associate religion with rigid dogmatism, blind superstition, empty ritual, hypocrisy, and with self-serving, even exploitative, bureaucracies and institutions. And indeed throughout history religious individuals and groups have committed in the name of religion every stupidity and atrocity of which we human beings are capable.

But the original meanings of religion and of religious are quite distinct from the associations with which history and human frailty have burdened them. The ancestor of the term religion is the Latin word *religare*. This consists of the root *ligare*, "to connect," and the prefix *re*, "to do something again." A religion then is something which "reconnects" what is now separate but was once together. It is God (or the Universal Spirit) and the human soul which are separate and to be reconnected. Thus a religious ideology is one which affirms an Absolute Reality and a human spirit, and which understands their reunion to be the ultimate destiny of the human being.

A religion must include a practice as well as a theory. In addition to an ideology which asserts that the aim of human life is union with the transcendent, a religion must have practical means to accomplish this end. The activities which bring the individual spirit closer to the divine being can be called "spiritual—or religious—practices."

The various traditions, theistic and pantheistic, have developed many diverse religious practices. These include worship; meditation; prayer; chanting and singing; reading and recitation of sacred literature; acts of self-denial and asceticism; acts of charity and selfless service; and pilgrimage. Thus, in human culture, a wide range of activities are considered "religious practices." Among the Society of Friends, sitting together in silence for an hour is a religious practice. Among the mountain ascetics of Japan, standing under a waterfall in midwinter is a religious practice. In Tantric Buddhism, ritual sexual intercourse is a religious practice. (The line forms on the right!) In Shi'ite Islam, self-flagellation on the day of Imam Hussain's martyrdom is one. These and a myriad other activities have a common goal, to bring the individual into close relationship with the divine.

For a person with a religious ideology, spiritual practice is a natural and logical consequence of his belief. But it is also an existential necessity. Our "spiritual body" must be nourished and exercised just as our physical or intellectual body must be fed and stimulated to activity. To neglect it is to neglect a vital part of ourselves. To nourish, exercise, and thereby expand the spirit, on a regular, preferably daily basis, is necessary to our health and happiness.

This "spiritual life" is so crucial that it emerges even from atheistic ideologies. Marxist-Leninism for example denies both God and the human spirit. But in practice it presents the Communist Party and the State as an ersatz Absolute, and creates a godless "religious life" around it. This atheistic "religion" includes ceremonies of praise and commemoration (May Day, the anniversary of the Russian Revolution), the veneration of saints (Marx, Lenin), the visitation of "holy places" (Lenin's tomb and birthplace), and opportunities (many, in fact) for self-sacrifice. Scientism similarly posits scientific knowledge and technological progress as an Absolute. It canonizes those who have devoted themselves to it (through the Nobel Prizes and other honors) and makes dedication to this absolute a sacred act. Our need as human beings to be part of something greater, to transcend our ego and individuality, is a basic and powerful one. We can ignore it only at our peril.

Thus a spiritual practice must be part of any way of life which aims at the full and happy development of the human being. To be Macrobiotic, then, involves having a spiritual life.

One can do this in a variety of ways. One can, for example, join a religious group whose beliefs closely match one's own. One can join a Methodist church, a Conservative synagogue, or a Buddhist society. And one can worship, pray, meditate, in the ways prescribed. There are advantages to this. The various activities have been developed and refined over centuries. Having proven spiritually satisfying to many prior generations, they will probably also satisfy us. Also, in the communal activities, one enjoys the company and support of other people. The phenomenon of synergy deepens one's religious experience.

But one can create one's own spiritual practice. One can select activities from several religions. One may draw upon foreign and alien traditions. One can practice alone and/or in private. Religious activity does not have to be public, organized, and communal. Nor does it have to come from one sect or from our own religious tradition.

Many people look to religions other than their own for spiritual practices. This is perhaps not as necessary as may appear. Each religious tradition includes a wide range of practices even as it includes a wide range of beliefs. The ideologies within Christianity range from the semi-pantheistic ideas of the left-wing Unitarians to the strict theism of the conservative wing of the Roman Catholic church. Similarly, it includes many varieties of prayer, meditation, and worship. If we delve deeply into our own tradition we will probably discover the religious practices which will satisfy us.

I have a Jewish friend who at an early age completely disavowed his own tradition. He got very interested in Buddhism in college. He went to Thailand, studied the language, and lived in a monastery for several years. His particular interest was in techniques for developing mental concentration and moral compassion. Tiring of life in an alien if fascinating culture, he came home. He happened to read some books on Judaism and was amazed to find that his own tradition contained ideas and disciplines very similar to those he had studied in Thailand. The treasure we seek in the far corners of the earth may already be in our hand.

In any case, we are free to take our practices from a single religious tradition or from several; to look only within our own cultural and religious tradition or to draw on others as well; to join a religious group, or to remain unaffiliated; to worship, pray, and meditate with others or by ourselves. Whichever options we choose, it is important that we have personally meaningful religious practices. And it is important that we practice them "religiously," that is, with regularity and with enthusiasm. Spiritual life is not the special domain of clerics, saints, and would-be saints. It should be part of the daily activity of every human being.

Even a person without a religious world view can have a spiritual practice. Many forms of meditation require no belief in a transcendent reality or in the human soul. Theravada Buddhism, for example, involves a sophisticated system of meditation but does not affirm the existence of a metaphysical Absolute or of an enduring human soul. And even a busy person should have a religious practice. As Jesus said, "What does it profit a man if he gains the world and loses his own soul?"

There are a number of basic forms of spiritual practice. They are found in most or all of the religious traditions, theistic and pantheistic. Each affects and benefits our spiritual body in a particular manner. A well-rounded spiritual life might include several, many, or all of the following:

Formulation and Recitation of a Creed: The word "creed" comes from the Latin *credo*, "to believe." It means a clear, systematic statement of belief. The Nicean and the Apostle's Creeds, for example, contain the essential tenets of the Christian Church and are frequently and regularly repeated by the faithful. Repeating a creed, whether an official ecclesiastical one, or a statement of our own composition, reminds us what we believe about the transcendent, about ourselves, and our destiny.

Prayer: The word "prayer" comes from the Latin *precari*, "to entreat" or "to beg." Thus in the theistic religions it has come to refer usually to petitionary conversation with God. The person praying asks for something. This may be comfort, strength, help for another person, or a solid gold Cadillac. Petitionary prayer is helpful (especially when its request is a disinterested one), in that it orients the mind and soul toward the divine.

But prayer can be understood as any mental or verbal exercise in which the soul orients itself to the divine and speaks to God. Thus there are various types of prayer. Worshipful prayer expresses affection, devotion, respect, and thanksgiving toward the divine. Confessional prayer opens the inner heart and reveals one's doubts and transgressions, and seeks forgiveness. Prayer can be inward and silent or spoken aloud. It can be individual or communal, public or private.

Prayer is central in the theistic traditions. The orthodox Jew and the devout Christian begin, end, and punctuate their day with prayer. The Muslim prays formally five times each day, orienting himself to Mecca and accompanying his words of praise and confession with physical gestures of obeisance. And in the non-Western traditions, wherever there is an element of theism or polytheism, prayer is practiced. Thus in Hinduism, the faithful pray to Vishnu and Shiva as personalized manifestations of the impersonal Brahman. And in Mahayana Buddhism, the Buddha is understood to be a cosmic deity, and is approached with prayers of petition, worship, and confession.

Ritual: A ritual is a prescribed set of words, gestures, and actions, often involving the use of objects. Many rituals are simply prayers accompanied by gesture and action. Thus there are petitionary rituals in which the Absolute is approached and asked for something. There are also rituals of worship, in which the divine is praised, honored, adored. Most sabbath services are largely rituals of worship. There are also rituals of confession and penance. The Roman Catholic "confession," with its penance of words and gestures, is such a ritual.

There are also rituals of commemoration, such as the Christian Eucharist and the Jewish Seder, in which an event is remembered and re-enacted. And there are rituals of sanctification, such as an ordination or marriage, in which a person, relationship, object, or place is "made holy."

Because ritual involves spoken words, gestures, actions, and objects, it is physically real. It provides perhaps a more powerful experience than silent or even spoken prayer. In the Seder, the Jew experiences Yahweh's liberation of His people from bondage in Egypt. In the Eucharist, the Christian encounters the suffering of Christ on the cross and the forgiveness and grace that suffering made possible. The Hindu in the *puja*, or "ritual of devotion," expresses his love of the deity by pouring offerings of water, milk, and melted butter over its image or symbol. Thus rituals make the experience of the sacred immediate, concrete, and powerful.

Meditation: Meditation is a silent looking inward. It involves the withdrawal of the senses from external stimulation and the focusing and stilling of the mind. The human soul is like a jewel lying on the bottom of a muddy pool. Meditation clears the water of the pool (our psyche) and allows us to clearly see and experience our soul. It also provides a quiet space for the presence and voice of God to enter.

There are different types of meditation. Most involve sitting

in an upright posture (the spine and head are the antennae of
the human body, able to attract and take in the energy of the
divine), with the eyes totally or partially closed. Some use an aid
to achieving concentration. This may be a physical object (such
as a lighted candle placed before one); a mental image; a paradoxical problem (such as the *koan* used in Soto Zen meditation);
or an inwardly repeated sound (such as the *mantra* of Transcendental Meditation). Some rely only on the mind itself to create
a state of "emptiness."

As a spiritual practice, meditation is more widely used perhaps
in the pantheistic than in the theistic traditions. But there are
Christian, Jewish, and Muslim forms of meditation as there are
Hindu, Buddhist, and Taoist forms. In each, the individual
orients himself to the divine.

Chanting: The vocal repetition of sacred syllables, phrases, or
passages in a rhythmic manner is a religious practice common
all over the world. According to Hindu thought there are seven
energy centers in the body, ranging from the sexual in the pubic
area to the spiritual at the top of the head. Each *chakra*, or
"wheel of energy," responds to stimulation by a particular wave
length of energy. A sacred syllable like AUM, or a phrase like
Ave Maria gratia plena, "Hail Mary full of grace," by virtue of
its sound and its meaning, affects the highest (spiritual) chakra.
Chanting thus can awaken and strengthen the spiritual body.
Chanting can be understood as an active and vocal form of
meditation.

Listening to and Performing Sacred Music: Music which has
been created by a person with spiritual awareness, and with
a spiritual purpose in mind, has, as does a mantra, a religious
power. It can nourish and activate the spirit of those who perform it and those who listen to it. Until the modern era, most
music had a direct or indirect religious intent. The aim of a Bach
cantata, an oratorio by Handel, and of a classical Indian *raga* is
to lift performers and audience alike out of the temporal and
mundane world into the realm of the infinite and eternal. In some

cultures, dance also has a sacred function. The whirling dance of the Sufis for example is meant to bring the dervish into contact with Allah.

The Contemplation of Religious Art: A painting, sculpture, or building created with spiritual intent by a religious person also has the power to transform and elevate consciousness. All cultures have realized this, and have used the pictorial and plastic arts as tools for spiritual development. In Tantric Buddhism, *mandalas*, or pictorial representations of the universe, are used as an object of meditation. In the Greek Orthodox Church, ikons or images of Christ, Mary, and the saints, are used in prayer and meditation. And of course the Roman Catholic Church, understanding the power of art to nourish the human spirit, has over the centuries been the West's greatest patron of painting, sculpture, and architecture. If we really take time to study and contemplate a sacred work, we take in and are transformed by its spiritual quality.

The Reading, Study, Recitation, and Memorization of Sacred Scriptures: Sacred scriptures contain in their sounds, images, and ideas, powerful spiritual energy. Thus to read, study, recite, and memorize holy literature is to approach the divine. Every literate religious tradition has used its sacred writings in spiritual practice. And nonliterate cultures, whose sacred traditions are preserved orally (usually in the form of myths), have used these in the same way.

In Judaism, for example, the study of the Torah and Talmud are at the center of religious life. Among Muslims, the memorization of the entire Koran, a book of about three hundred pages, is an important act of piety. In Buddhism, the recitation (and also the copying by hand) of the Heart Sutra is a common spiritual practice. Many Christians read daily from their Scriptures.

Fasting and Other Forms of Abstinence: Abstention from food for a specific period has been used as a spiritual practice in almost every culture and period. Fasting cuts a primary bond with the relative material world. It helps us see our own spiritual nature and to be open to divine inspiration. George Ohsawa compared the human organism to a radio receiver able to pick up various vibrations. And he said that to fast is to clean this receiver and to orient its antennae towards the Infinite. Hence the fasting person can pick up the most ethereal and spiritual of the vibrations in the universe. Many of the great religious figures in human history, including Moses, Gautama, Jesus, and Mohammad, fasted prior to their key spiritual experiences.

A fast of even one or several days can be beneficial. At the very least, it makes us grateful for the gift of food and of life. At one time the Lenten period was a time of fasting for Christians. Jews abstain from food on Yom Kippur, the day of atonement. Each year Muslims fast, abstaining from food and drink during daylight hours for the month of Ramadan.

Abstinence from other common and habitual activities also has been observed for spiritual ends. Celibacy, either temporary or lifelong, is practiced in many cultures. Like fasting, this practice severs a strong bond to the physical world and allows one to focus on the life of the spirit. Muslims are celibate during their pilgrimage to the holy city of Mecca. In Buddhism and Christianity, those who wish to devote themselves to spiritual development—priests, monks, and nuns—may observe a lifelong sexual abstinence.

Mahatma Gandhi practiced "verbal fasting." One day a week he would refrain from speaking. He said that this practice freed him from a host of distractions; allowed him to focus his energy; and brought him in contact with his inner spirit. The monks of the Trappist order take a vow of silence in addition to the usual vows of poverty, celibacy, and obedience.

The "social fast," is an intentional withdrawal from all social contact and worldly involvement for a specific period. It can be observed at points of transition (just before marriage or upon retirement), in moments of personal crisis, or on a regular, perhaps annual basis. Such a retreat allows us to survey our lives and ourselves objectively, and to look within for spiritual

216

strength. In Japan, many common citizens—engineers, house-
wives, laborers—periodically spend a week or more in a monastery or *dojo* (place for spiritual training).

Observance of the Sabbath: While the Sabbath is a day of
"rest," it need not be a day of inactivity. A respite from the
cares and distractions of the world, it is also an opportunity to
nourish our spirit. Prayer, ritual, music, are all as important to
the Sabbath as the Sunday paper and the professional football
game.

Holidays, like the Sabbath, are "holy days" and can be used
for spiritual as well as recreational ends. Prayer, ritual, meditation, are as appropriate on national holidays, birthdays, on New
Year's day, and the first day of Spring, as on Yom Kippur and
Christmas. Each special day has a meaing and significance which
should be noted, understood, and experienced. The experience
and the expression of gratitude for the blessing of life, rather
than the consumption of a dead turkey, lies at the heart of
Thanksgiving Day.

Acts of Charity and Selfless Service: Most of our actions arise
from self-interest. We do them because they benefit us or benefit
people with whom we closely identify—family members, spouse,
children, and friends. This is human and natural. However, we
are capable also of acts of charity. These do not directly or
obviously benefit us or anyone close to us. They may in fact
inconvenience or deprive us. Most religions have recognized
such acts as essential to spiritual development.

Giving to charitable or religious institutions, helping the poor
and disadvantaged, even offering a word of kindness to a
stranger (or enemy) all diminish the power of the ego, and
nourish the spirit. The Muslim is encouraged to give a fortieth
of his total wealth annually to the care of the poor. And in
Judaism and Christianity, great value is placed on acts of compassion and selfless service. *Tithing*, or giving one-tenth of one's
income to the poor or to the Church, is considered a mark of
the devout Christian. In Buddhism, *karuna* or a disinterested

compassion which issues in acts of help and kindness, is the
highest virtue. And in Hinduism, *karma yoga*, "the path of
selfless acts," is understood as essential to spiritual development.

Pilgrimage: Certain places possess special spiritual power.
They do so because of geographical influences and/or because of
what human beings have done there. For example, in many
cultures, mountain tops are considered spiritually potent. Pointing
to the heavens, they act as antennae for the energy of the divine.
Places where "ley lines" (the energy pathways which cover the
earth's surface) intersect also are special. If at such an intersection human activity has further sanctified the ground, then it
possesses a very strong energy. In Great Britain and elsewhere
in Europe, monuments, cathedrals and monasteries (Stonehenge,
Chartres, Mont-St.-Michel) are believed to be located on cross-
ings of the ley lines. There the worship and the lives of holy
people through the centuries have created a powerful resource
of sacred energy.

To travel to a holy place with a spiritual intent, to pray,
meditate, and perform rituals there, is to partake of its power.
Hence Jews go to the Wailing Wall in Jerusalem, Christians to
Bethlehem, Rome, and Canterbury, Muslims to Mecca, Buddhists to Bodhgaya, the Japanese to Ise, and members of every
other religion to their particular holy places.

There are, then, many forms of spiritual activity. These can be
carried out by the individual, by a family group, or by a larger
congregation. They can be observed hourly, daily, weekly, or
annually. They can be observed according to the prescribed
tradition of a certain faith, or according to one's own inclination. These religious practices all nourish and exercise the spiritual body, helping it however slightly, to draw nearer to the
transcendent.

Our spiritual life does not benefit only our spiritual body.
Each activity influences one or more of our other bodies as
well. Fasting purifies the physical self as well as our spiritual
self. The appreciation of religious music and art nourishes our

218

aesthetic sense. Prayer and meditation calm the emotions. Study of sacred texts exercises the mind and our ideological faculty. Acts of selfless service refine our ethical awareness. A pilgrimage to a distant shrine teaches us much about the world and the people in it. In fact, no activity is purely spiritual.

The converse of this statement is also true. All activities are ultimately spiritual. Each action in each dimension of our life— physical, aesthetic, emotional, intellectual, social, and ideological—affects our spiritual body. Everything we think, do, and say either injures or benefits our spirit in its progress toward union with the Absolute. Thus, our spiritual life requires (and includes):

- A whole foods, natural diet, good water, good air, natural light, exercise, natural fibre clothing.
- An aesthetically pleasing environment and creative artistic activity.
- Self-acceptance, a satisfying vocation, loving relationships with friends and family, full emotional expression, a sense of community, and play.
- A vital intellectual life and positive habits of mind.
- A social life in which the laws of reciprocity, of ahimsa, and of love are manifest in every thought, word, and action.
- A serious, continuous attempt to understand the universe and our place in it and to express our beliefs coherently and systematically.

In other words, whatever contributes to our health in any dimension of life, contributes to our spiritual health. Everything we do then can be "spiritual" or "religious."

Since the introduction of Macrobiotics in the West, the question has often been raised: Is Macrobiotics a religion?

Macrobiotics is not a religion in the way that Roman Catholicism, Lutheranism, Islam, and Buddhism are religions. It has no specific, generally accepted statement of principles and beliefs. Despite the insightful brilliance of my "artichoke theory," only my dog and I agree that it captures the true essence of

Macrobiotics. Macrobiotics has no churches, clergy, rituals, or ecclesiastical organization. In fact, it has little organization at all. Its main concern seems to be with physical health. It gives only modest attention to overtly "spiritual" concerns.

The idea that each human being has a grand and beautiful destiny, however, lies at the base of Macrobiotics. And all its practices aim at the realization of that destiny. Ultimately, Macrobiotics seeks the union of the individual with the transcendent. If religion, in its pure sense, is the reconnection of the human and the divine, then Macrobiotics, both in its ideology and way of life, is a "religion."

9. Illness and Healing

A wise man should consider that health is the
greatest of blessings, and learn by his own thought
how to derive benefit from his illnesses.
                          Hippocrates (c. 460–400 B.C.)

He delivers the afflicted by their affliction, and opens
their ear by diversity.
                          The Book of Job, 36: 15

Thus far we have considered health from a positive viewpoint.
We have defined it as the full, positive functioning of each of
our bodies—from physical to spiritual—and we have made
practical suggestions for nourishing and exercising each. We
have said little about illness, its cause or its cure.

But to speak of health is also to speak of illness. The two are
opposite and complementary realities. Illness is the absence of
health. Its cause is the lack of those factors necessary for health.
And its cure must involve the cultivation of those same factors.

As health is the full, dynamic functioning of our various
bodies, illness is their partial or imperfect functioning. In each
body, sickness manifests in a different way.

In the physical body, sickness is pain, biochemical and biomechanical dysfunction, low and inconsistent energy, poor
appetite for food and sex, and poor sleep.

In the aesthetic body, it is an inability to perceive and experience the beauty which characterizes the natural world and much
of the human-made world. It is also an inability to express one's
own creative instincts in a coherent and satisfying manner.

In the emotional body, it is a predominance (both in dura-
tion and intensity) of unpleasant and painful emotions. In emotional illness, negative affects such as fear, anxiety, sadness,
anger, jealousy, and remorse are more intense and long lasting
than the positive affects.

In the intellectual body, illness is a lack of curiosity about the

world and an underdevelopment of the mental abilities: observation, memory, reasoning, comprehension, and imagination.
Also, it is the dominance of negative, inhibiting, and destructive mental attitudes over positive ones.

In the social or moral body, it is the rule of self-interest rather than of kindness and compassion in relations with other human beings, with animals and plants, and with inanimate nature.

In the ideological body, sickness is an indifference to the basic questions concerning the universe and human life, and a resulting lack of a carefully considered and systematic view of the world.

In the spiritual body, it is the alienation, ennui, and despair which result from living in a universe perceived and experienced as devoid of meaning.

Sometimes illness has a single, specific cause, or seems to. A man falls on an icy sidewalk and breaks his leg. A woman is sexually assaulted and develops emotional problems. In such cases the illness manifests primarily in the body most directly affected. Though he may get depressed about his immobility, the man's primary concern is his painful, nonfunctioning leg.
Though she may develop insomnia as a side effect, the woman is troubled mostly by emotional trauma.

For a one-dimensional illness a focused therapy will work.
If the man's leg is splinted, and he spends three weeks in bed he should be back to his normal condition. If the woman receives counseling, is able to relive her experience and to release the trauma associated with it, she too should return to her prior condition. Thus an illness with a single cause, likely has a single manifestation, and will respond to a one-dimensional treatment.

However, many, perhaps most sicknesses, are complex in cause and in manifestation. They result from several factors, not just a single one. And while they affect one area most obviously, they actually affect several or even all of our bodies. And their cure must involve a multi-dimensional therapy.

In a typical case of stomach ulcers, for example, the patient consumes much sweets, fatty foods, coffee, alcohol, and other things which directly irritate the stomach. But also he is under great emotional and psychological stress. His job is at risk; his marriage is a difficult one; he has been involved in some illicit financial dealings. The worry, unhappiness, and guilt affects his ulcer directly, by causing excessive flow of digestive juices, and indirectly, by influencing his eating habits. He drowns his sorrows in sweets, alcohol, and overeating. Thus his job situation, his marriage, and his ethical problems are as much a cause of his sickness as is his diet.

And actually the ulcers are not his sickness. They are only its most obvious manifestation. His emotional and moral bodies are equally ill. The dysfunctions in the several areas form a syndrome of interrelated symptoms, which are all equally important.

In "non-physical" sicknesses also, the causes and the manifestations usually are complex. *Agoraphobia*, for example, is an unreasoning and extreme fear of public places. It primarily afflicts women. A person with agoraphobia may be terrified to leave her house, and even in a supermarket may be overcome with fear. In a typical case, emotional factors certainly are crucial. Because of a cruel and domineering father, the woman may be possessed by guilt and by a sense of personal inadequacy. But other life factors are also contributing to her sensitivity and anxiety. She eats a junk-food diet of crackers, potato chips, ice cream, and Coca Cola, which predisposes her to hypoglycemia. She leads a sedentary and indoor life. Indifferent to religion, she has never dealt with the serious issues of existence. Nor does she have any spiritual practice to enrich her life. Thus, there are physical, ideological, and spiritual causes for her "emotional illness." And her illness is not only an emotional one. In her physical, ideological, and spiritual bodies there are simultaneous and interrelated problems.

When the causes and manifestations of a sickness are complex, the therapy must be multi-dimensional. It must seek to eliminate all of the causes and it must treat each of the bodies involved. A one-dimensional therapy directed at the most obvious symptom will give some relief. But it will be only a partial and temporary relief. The problems in the other areas, while lessened, will persist. And since the secondary and underlying causes remain, even the main symptom eventually will reoccur, in its old or perhaps in a new form.

If the stomach-ulcer patient receives medication, has an operation, or changes his diet, his symptoms probably will disappear. But if nothing is done to change his professional and marital situation, and to deal with his guilt, he will continue to suffer on the emotional and moral levels. He will still be "sick." He may be able to hold to a moderate and balanced diet—which is very difficult if one is emotionally and psychologically stressed. But even if he does, in time those non-physical problems will manifest on the physical level as ulcers again, or as migraine headaches, or as something else.

Similarly, the agoraphobe might be helped by psychological counseling, and she might become able to go again into public. But this cure also will be limited and temporary. Her physical and other problems will persist and in time will issue in the same or another emotional illness.

For a full and lasting cure, especially of a chronic or serious illness, a holistic, multi-dimensional approach is necessary. This approach is based on the fact that all the bodies are profoundly interrelated, that each is constantly affecting and being affected by all the others. It involves a careful consideration and diagnosis of each body, not just the one most obviously afflicted. And it involves the strengthening and treatment of each in a way appropriate to it.

For the stomach-ulcer patient, a multi-factor approach, in addition to dietary changes, would include marital counseling, and perhaps a vocational change. It would also involve a clearing of the patient's conscience, perhaps through a process of confession, apology, and penance. For the agoraphobe, a holistic therapy, in addition to emotional counseling, would include a whole-foods diet, and regular outdoor exercise. It might comprise, as well, serious consideration of ideological issues and perhaps some basic spiritual practice, such as meditation or volunteer charity work.

A true holistic diagnosis requires time, patience, and rare

insight. A holistic treatment also requires time and patience, and competence in (or at least familarity with) a wide variety of therapies and measures. The question arises: "To whom can one go for such diagnosis and treatment?"

Medical practitioners in the West fall into two broad categories, allopathic and "alternative." Allopathy has been the dominant or standard system of medicine for about the past eighty years. "Alternative" medicine is everything other than allopathy. Thus it includes acupuncture, aromatherapy, chiropractic, homeopathy, naturopathy, Macrobiotics, Christian Science, and a variety of other therapies.

Allopathic medicine is based on three principles:

1. The human body is a biological machine.
2. The primary causes of disease are the invasion of the body by pathogenic organisms, such as viruses and bacteria, and the chemical or mechanical breakdown of the body.
3. Medical procedures should destroy pathogens (through antagonistic or allopathic medications); should redress chemical imbalances (also through medication); should repair mechanical problems (through surgery); and if it cannot eliminate the cause of an illness, should through medication and/or surgery eliminate or mask its symptoms.

Allopathic medicine tends to be analytical and symptomatic. It views the physical body in isolation from the rest of the human organism, and it even views different parts of the body in isolation from the rest of the body. Thus it has engendered a vast and complex system of specialists, who focus on one part of the body and/or on one particular disease. There are heart specialists, foot specialists, cancer specialists, and AIDS specialists. Most of the procedures of allopathic medicine are invasive. They often have serious adverse effects, and while they eliminate the symptoms, they may not remove the underlying cause of the problem.

Allopathic medicine is excellent in dealing with acute and emergency conditions (broken bones, gunshot wounds, and complications in childbirth), with much infectious disease and with some biomechanical problems. In many circumstances, its procedures are faster, more efficient, and more certain than anything alternative medicine can offer. Allopathic medicine is a resource, which even the most ardent Macrobiotic person can and should use when appropriate.

For example, one evening I received a phone call from a young Macrobiotic woman. She was very distressed and told me that her boyfriend was in a bad way. His left testicle was swollen to the size of a grapefruit. On questioning her, I learned that this swollen testicle was his only one. He had lost the other in a motorcycle accident a few years back. As a bicycle tour leader, I happen to know a bit about his condition which often results from a cycling accident. So I said to her:

"My dear friend, take yourself and your boyfriend, and his sole remaining testicle, and go as fast as you can to the emergency room of the nearest hospital."

"Don't you think a tofu plaster might help?" she asked in desperation.

"If a distended testicle is not drained within four hours," I replied, "it starts to die. Now there is a time for tofu plasters and there is a time for standard emergency medical attention. This is not a time for tofu!"

Allopathic medicine is by nature analytical and symptomatic. Nevertheless, there are physicians who view the body as an integrated phenomenon (not as the aggregation of separate parts) and who view physical health as deeply related to emotional and mental health. There are, in other words, holistically inclined medical doctors. These include General Practitioners who have realized that to understand a person's illness you must understand his entire life. These also include physicians (many younger ones among them) who have been influenced by the holistic movement and/or by recent discoveries of medical research. These doctors are aware of the importance of diet and exercise in the prevention and cure of disease. They are aware also of the role of emotions and mental attitudes in affecting our ability to resist disease and to recover from it. Relatively speaking, however, such holistic physicians are still few in number. The approach of the typical doctor is analytical, and his treatments are likely to be invasive and radical.

Many of the alternative therapies are founded on a holistic view of the human organism. Traditional Chinese Medicine, which includes acupuncture, herbal medicine, and certain types of massage, for example, is based on an integrated view of the human being. Naturopathy, homeopathy, chiropractic, osteopathy, and most of the host of other alternative therapies also affirm the unity of body, mind, and spirit. Thus, one is more likely to find a holistic therapist among alternative practitioners.

However, it is still very difficult. Many alternative therapists, despite a theoretical holism, are actually very narrow in their diagnoses and in their treatments. There are chiropractors who see all problems as the result of spinal subluxation alone, and use nothing other than spinal adjustment. There are massage therapists who see all problems as the result of muscle imbalance and use only muscle therapy. There are acupuncturists who see all ailments as resulting from an imbalance of Ch'i flow. They use needles to correct this and thus relieve immediate discomfort and pain. But they disregard other causal factors and other therapies. Therefore one can't assume that every alternative practitioner is necessarily holistic. Copies of *Rolling Stone* and *Vegetarian Times* in the waiting room, Jackson Browne on the stereo, and a Tibetan mandala on the wall behind the receptionist, doth not a holistic therapist make.

Besides, although a therapist may have a holistic viewpoint, he may not make full use of it in practice. It takes time and patience to carefully work through all the dimensions of an individual's life. It takes a wide knowledge and experience to offer advice or treatment for emotional, psychological, and spiritual problems. A well-intentioned practitioner may know that emotional life and habits of mind are important factors in a patient's condition. He may however lack the time and/or confidence to get involved in these other areas. So in the thirty minutes or hour allotted to each patient, the acupuncturist, chiropractor, or massage therapist does what he knows how to do, recommends what he can, and hoping for the best, goes on to the next patient.

With a sickness whose cause and manifestation are one-dimensional this may suffice. A muscle, painful after exposure to damp and cold, probably will respond to an acupuncture treatment which renews Ch'i flow in the area. A vertebrae out of alignment because of a car accident may be corrected by spinal manipulation alone. The trauma occasioned by the death of a spouse or child can be helped just by counseling and trauma-release therapy.

But chronic and serious conditions need more. These require a total diagnosis, one that looks deeply at every aspect of a person's life, from physical to spiritual, and that identifies problem areas in each. And chronic and serious conditions require a complex and intense therapy which involves basic changes in each area of life. An effective and lasting cure for a deep illness may require many or all of the following:

- Dietary change; a new source of drinking water; a physical exercise program; a new wardrobe; changes in one's living and working environment; new patterns of relaxation, rest, and sleep.
- A new interior design for one's home; purging of excess possessions; new tastes in music and art; courses in ceramics, art, music, or dance.
- A new sense of self-acceptance and self-worth; a new and satisfying vocation; deepened relationships with family and friends; heightened community involvement and learning to play.
- Resumption or continuation of academic education; a new, intellectually challenging hobby; a systematic review and change of one's habits of mind.
- Reevaluation of moral and ethical life, leading to new ways of relating to other people, animals, plants, and the natural world.

- Active and careful consideration of the basic questions of human existence, and the formulation of a personal ideology.
- Development of a spiritual practice, including worship, meditation, prayer, and selfless service.

Such changes cannot be affected by a practitioner in thirty minutes or an hour. They require long, hard, and unremitting effort by the person himself.

Thus, from even the most gifted holistic healer, alternative or allopathic, we can expect only limited help. He may be able to diagnose us completely. He may be able to give us some relief from our most troublesome symptoms. He may be able to recommend many of the other changes necessary to cure us totally. But even if he can do all this (which is very difficult and very unlikely), he cannot carry out the changes necessary to our cure. In the end, our therapy and cure rests with us. Only we can do those things which will render our various bodies, and our total being, "whole."

Thus we are our own best physician. Certainly a health professional's diagnosis and prescription can be helpful. But the fullest diagnosis and prescription comes from within. Only we know ourselves well enough, and have sufficient time and interest to examine, with the necessary care, every aspect of our life. Only we can know how each area—physical, aesthetic, emotional, intellectual, social, ideological, and spiritual—needs to be changed. And certainly a health professional's treatments can be helpful. But only we can make the changes in ourselves and in our way of life that will affect a real cure. We must be chief physician as well as patient. Upon us all, rests the Gospel injunction, "Physician, heal thyself!"

I have learned this the hard way. I am blessed with a strong physical constitution. My parents both came from sturdy German peasant stock. My father lived to eighty-four and was quite active and healthy until the last two years of his life. My mother is alive and vigorous at eighty. I have a natural love of exercise and the outdoors and have always indulged this. Also, I discovered Macrobiotics at age twenty-one, before discovering drugs, alcohol, and other common forms of abuse. For these reasons I have enjoyed good health throughout my life. I have had no serious illness and can count on my fingers the days spent in bed because of illness.

About four years ago, made proud by this fact, I began giving lectures on the topic, "Macrobiotics Beyond Food." These were well-received and I got the idea of writing a book based on the material. About eighteen months ago I signed a contract with Japan Publications and began working on this book. Of course, God, or the Tao or whoever or whatever runs the show is a master of irony and the practical joke. So just as I was beginning my treatise on health, I got sick!

For several years I had been conscious of a slight stiffness in my neck. This condition got worse when I did a lot of bicycling, rock climbing, hiking with a heavy pack, or sitting at a desk. Suddenly it began to bother me a great deal.

I consulted a chiropractor, who took X-rays and said that several cervical vertebrae were out of alignment. He did an adjustment which relieved the tension in my neck and shoulders. Unfortunately, this adjustment did not hold. I felt fine for a few days, but then the vertebrae again slipped out, and the stiffness and tension returned. A second adjustment also lasted a short time. The pattern continued. Each time the neck "went out" the severity of the symptoms increased. Soon I was dealing with a painful tension all through my neck and upper back, which sapped my physical, emotional, and psychological energy.

The chiropractor was a well-meaning and compassionate person with a holistic outlook. And his adjustments did give me some temporary relief. But we did not seem to be making progress and I couldn't afford thirty dollar sessions indefinitely. So I began to look elsewhere for help.

Over the next year I consulted in turn a medical doctor, an osteopathic doctor, a nutritional counselor, and several acupuncturists and massage therapists. They all agreed that the immediate cause was muscular, that my neck and shoulder muscles were tense and spastic and were pulling the vertebrae

out of alignment. Each had a different view of the underlying
cause and of the best treatment. Happy at any promise of relief,
I went along with most of the recommended therapies. I adjusted my diet, took vitamin and mineral supplements, did
"corrective exercises," was massaged, needled, and even fitted
out with magnets. Each approach afforded some relief, but it
was always partial and/or temporary. While my conditions
generally improved, I was still afflicted and did not know how
to cure my affliction. I was desperate.

Throughout this ordeal, I had maintained the hope that the
problem was physical and superficial, and that the right practitioner would magically massage or needle it away. I had resisted
the idea that it was connected to the rest of my life, and would
require major changes to cure. But I could ignore this no longer.
Most of the therapists had mentioned "stress" as a possible
underlying factor. Stress of course is a pretty broad term. I knew
though I had to find out what it meant in relation to me and
to my own condition. Otherwise, I would never get better.

So I began to review each aspect of my life. I looked at my
physical, aesthetic, emotional, intellectual, social, ideological,
and spiritual bodies. I tried to discover sources of stress in each.
Soon a number of factors, which a typical diagnosis probably
would not uncover and which a typical therapy could do little
to treat, became apparent. These included, among many others,
the facts that:

- I was in a relationship with a woman which was causing us
  both much emotional turmoil.
- I had not fully dealt with the death of my father two years
  previous.
- I was leading a hyperactive, hyper-mobile life which
  precluded deep personal and community attachments.
- I was in an occupation which often involves more physical
  and psychic strain than I can easily deal with.
- Although a religious person, I had neglected my spiritual
  practice for a long time.

I realized that a simple diet, improved posture, stretching exercises, muscle therapy, and acupuncture treatments would all help my neck problem. But I also realized that to cure it I would have to deal with the other problems in my life. So I began to deal seriously and honestly with the problems in my relationship. I confronted and released my feelings regarding my father's death. I began to think of ways to slow down and enrich my life. I started to arrange work obligations to avoid stress for extended periods. And I have begun to set aside time for spiritual practice.

This kind of healing process is long and difficult. It requires patience, courage, willingness to take risks, and will-power. And I must confess that even as I write the last chapters of this book on health, I am still in the midst of it.

But such healing is essential to our growth and development. Each sickness is really a great blessing. It is a loving reminder from God and nature that we must live according to His will and its laws. And illness is an opportunity to examine each part of our lives and to make it and ourselves more whole. If we use this reminder and this opportunity well we can emerge stronger, wiser, more compassionate and healthy than we were before.

Conclusion

It was the best of times, it was the worst of times.
Charles Dickens (1812–1870)

Today we citizens of the industrial West live in a paradoxical situation. In many ways we are greatly blessed, perhaps more so than any people in history. We enjoy great material wealth. In terms of food, clothing, housing, means of transportation, conveniences and comforts, information, entertainment, and education, we are rich, very rich. And we enjoy near total individual, political, and religious freedom.

But in other ways we are severely disadvantaged. We have paid a price for this abundance and freedom. Many of those things essential to human health and happiness, which were part of traditional, pre-industrial life, have disappeared or at least have become difficult to obtain. And in their stead we have things which undermine, sometimes obviously and directly, sometimes insidiously, our health and well-being.

Thus while we need simple, pure, wholesome foods, we have a cornucopia of refined and industrially processed products. Though these are beautifully packaged, convenient, and often delicious, they do not fully nourish or sustain life.

While we need clean water, fresh air, natural light, we have polluted water and air, and artificial light. While we need contact with the wholesome energies of earth and heaven, we are insulated from these and instead are surrounded by potentially dangerous energies.

While our eyes hunger for the beauty of trees, plants, flowers, and streams, we live in a morass of tract homes, shopping malls, expressways, parking lots, and mammoth buildings of concrete and glass. And while our ears hunger for the gentle sounds of nature and for her silences, we are surrounded by a ceaseless cacophony of mechanical and electronic noise.

While we need a human pace of life and ample rest and relaxation, we live at a frenetic speed, rushing here and there, driven by our machines even in times of leisure.

While we need to sing and dance and play, we sit and watch the flickering image of others dancing, singing, and playing.

While we need the love and support of family, friends, and community, we often find ourselves alone or in the company of strangers. The rambling home which sheltered three generations of family has been converted into a condominium of studio and one-bedroom apartments.

While we need vocations which are creative and meaningful, we have more and more jobs which are mechanical and in which effort and product are unconnected.

While we need intellectual stimulation and challenge, we have instead an endless flood of trivial and lobotomizing media entertainment. The most taxing intellectual act of our time, thanks to the home VCR, has become keeping track of the movies we have not yet seen.

While we need clear ethical and moral standards by which to guide our life, we have instead a self-serving moral relativism. And while we need examples of virtue to help us in the awesome task of becoming "good" human beings, we are surrounded by images of self-indulgence, greed, and dishonesty.

While we need inspiration to grapple with the serious issues of life and to formulate a clear world view, we instead get encouragement to consume and to borrow.

While we need direction and instruction in developing a satisfying spiritual life, we have the superficiality and excesses of "TV evangelism."

And while we need a holistic, integrative, and patient-centered approach to healing, we have instead a medical system which is analytical and symptomatic and which encourages our dependency upon it.

These are generalizations of course, and harsh ones. The actual situation varies from place to place, and it is always changing. In some ways it is getting better. Air pollution levels, for example, are decreasing in certain areas. In other ways, it is getting worse. We are surrounded by and dependent on more and more electronic and mechanical devices. In any case, to be a healthy and happy human being today is a real challenge. And it is not surprising that despite the billions of dollars spent on health care we are afflicted with epidemic rates of heart disease, cancer, AIDS, sterility, mental illness, divorce, crime, and other symptoms of individual, family, and social dissolution.

It is in fact amazing that we survive and thrive as well as we do. This is a tribute to the flexibility and durability of the human body, mind, and spirit. It is a tribute as well to the vitality of our ancestors which has been passed down to us, albeit in diluted form.

Despite the obstacles with which we have surrounded ourselves, it is possible today to enjoy health and well-being. Perfect health of course is an ideal. When we have fully developed each of our bodies, from physical to spiritual, we will be in heaven. But meanwhile, we can be constantly drawing nearer to that ideal of wholeness. And the difficulties which we encounter on route will increase our strength and flexibility and deepen our understanding.

The Macrobiotic way of life is a path towards health. It involves eating a diet of wholesome, ecological foods. It includes also nourishing the body with good water, air, and energy, and exercising and resting it properly.

The Macrobiotic way of life includes also the nourishment and exercise of each of the other human bodies—aesthetic, emotional, intellectual, social, ideological, and spiritual. The wholeness of each is vitally important and we must cultivate them all with equal care and energy.

This book is a tentative and incomplete attempt to explore the fullness of the *Macrobiotic Way of Life*. It has discussed various ways to cultivate the health of our various bodies. But it has touched only a few of the things possible and necessary. Nevertheless, I hope that it has been helpful. I hope also that it has stimulated the readers' own insights and discoveries. I await your comments, suggestions, and additions, humbly and with anticipation. We are travelers on this road together. I wish you well.

Bibliography

Dadd, Deborah Lee. *Non Toxic and Natural*, Jeremy Tarcher, Los Angeles, 1984
———. *The Non-Toxic Home*, Tarcher, L. A., 1986

Zamm, Alfred. *Why Your House May Endanger Your Health*, Simon and Schuster, 1980.

Soyka, Fred. *The Ion Effect*, Bantam Books, 1978

Garvey, Jack. *The Five Phases of Food*, Well-Being Books, 1985

Ott, John, Dr. *Health and Light*, Bantam Books, 1979

Tame, Michael. *The Secret Power of Music*, Inner traditions, Rochester, Vermont, 1986.

Tompkin, Peter, Dr. *The Secret Life of Plants*, Harper and Row, 1973

Ineson, John. *The Way of Life; Macrobiotics and the Spirit of Christianity*, Japan Publications, 1986

Aihara, Herman. *Learning From Salmon*, GOMF Press, Oroville, CA. 1984

Index